FROM STRESSED TO BLESSED

overcoming anxiety and low mood
with minor lifestyle changes

Anne Cross

Bsc Nutritional Medicine Bsc Occupational Therapy

The contents of this book have been written for education and information purposes only. It is not intended to serve as a substitute for medical advice. Please consult a qualified medical practitioner or other health professional if you have any queries or concerns regarding any health issues you may have. The author or publisher accept no responsibility for the reader choosing to self prescribe with any listed supplements, suggested techniques or nutrition changes as discussed and outlined in this book.

Published by Anne Cross
First CreateSpace Edition 2017

Editor: Angela Clarence
Interior Design: Geoff Fisher
Cover design: Cassia Friello
Illustrations: Cassia Friello

www.annecrossnutrition.co.uk

CONTENTS

I dedicate this book to my family.

Thanks to you mum and dad for loving me, for always
being there for me, and for babysitting!

Thanks to my sister Julia for her support which helped give me the strength
to carry on in my darkest moments, and for banter at the gym!

Thanks to you my calm and lovely husband John for always
accepting me for me.

Thanks to my beautiful daughter who brings joy, chaos
and love into my life.

And thanks to my in-laws Anne and Mark Bisset for their
kindness, a listening ear and an open house.

INTRODUCTION

THE aim of the book is to help you become more conscious of how food, lifestyle, thoughts, and emotions can affect physical and mental wellbeing. We are all presented with challenges in life, and mine led to both mental and physical breakdowns. I came to realise that hard times, whether caused by heartbreak or illness, are merely opportunities for growth and in my case, this led to a mind-blowing discovery - daily self-care - making small, ongoing lifestyle changes can transform the results of even the most devastating upsets and suffering.

While transformation takes time, making incremental changes in our food choices, exercise, sleep patterns and our thinking really work. It took me a while to realise that to get well – to become calm and present and positive about life - I had to practice and have patience - not my strongest attributes! If you want to be a good tennis player or piano player, you have to practice and so it is with working on oneself. Awareness, practice and patience get you there. APP - just a wee acronym I made up! Awareness, Practice, Patience!

For those of you who are struggling with physical and mental health problems, I hope that my experiences will give you hope. As well as igniting the understanding that we, ourselves, can take care of our health and healing; that some of my experiences, thoughts, feelings and awakenings that both hindered and helped my healing will resonate with you and help you to feel happier, healthier and more connected to yourself.

I write this with gratitude for my learning, which is ongoing, and with love for you in my heart. I believe that life is for living, but also for growing and learning. Developing awareness of our thoughts, responses and behaviour, is the first step in creating change and moving forward. No self-judgement needed!

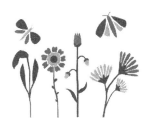

Chapter One

MY JOURNEY

I PROMISE this won`t be pages long.

As a happy, healthy child, I always felt loved. I enjoyed playing outside and was stoic in the face of the unexpected. On the way to hospital with a broken dislocated elbow, I remember cheerfully asking the teacher what football team he supported! I also remember the terrible disappointment that I wouldn't be able to play in the upcoming hockey match the following Saturday.

My mum who was a teacher and my dad who worked as an accountant always expected me to do well at school and although I put myself under pressure, studying hard to pass my exams, I wasn't quite up there with my school friends. When those friends continued their education to become doctors, lawyers, and accountants, I was eager to start earning and enjoying myself. I took a job in a bank and had a lot of fun in my late teens and early 20's although I probably drank too much. Then I failed my bank exams - four times! Finance wasn't for me. I had a feeling that I wanted to work with people, so I decided to go to college after all and studied Occupational Therapy. Determined to succeed I again put myself under pressure, qualified and entered a rewarding but challenging job in the Mental Health sector.

I continued to put myself under pressure – subconsciously determined to prove that I was worthy - both to my parents and myself. This ongoing stress began to show up in infections and viruses which were treated with antibiotics. I took time off to travel but roaming the world didn't solve my underlying subconscious problems, and I was eventually diagnosed with Chronic Fatigue Syndrome commonly called ME.

Unable to work, I moved back with my parents for a year to recover my strength. It was one of the hardest times of my life. I spent day after day after day in bed. I lost friends. I had no social life. I had no love life! Even taking a morning shower used every scrap of energy. Meanwhile, my sister was winning Tae Kwon Do medals and world titles, which added nothing to my feelings of self-worth!

Thank heavens I came under the care of a Doctor who had had ME himself. With his help and that of an energy therapist (thank you Zoe) plus a nutritionist and reflexologist (thank you beautiful May Anderson), I slowly began to recover my strength. Thank you, mum and dad, but also sorry. I was only meant to be home for a year, and it took nearly five!

The love of family, partner and friends are important healing components. I also noticed the impact that food and nutrition were making in supporting my healing journey. It sparked real interest, and during that period of recovery, I gained a BSc in Nutritional Medicine and began to rebuild my life. I joined a social group. I went walking. I was meeting lovely people, and even signed up to a dating site!

Unfortunately, the relationship that resulted broke up just as my maternal instinct kicked in. I didn't meet my partner John for another seven years, and it was another three years before we decided to have a baby when I was the ripe old age of 38. We tried for a couple of years but nothing happened even though all our tests showed positive, and I was using nutrition, supplements and other therapies. We had funds for one round of IVF, and I became pregnant but miscarried. The disappointment was tremendous, and when you miscarry, you can't help noticing that everyone else around you seems to be pregnant. However, three months later I became pregnant again, naturally! Was it the detox, the acupuncture, the self-connection course, or letting go a bit? Who knows!

I had Sophia (meaning Wisdom) aged 41, with an emergency C-section. Not quite the birth I had imagined (music, massage oils and measured breathing), but just two days after the birth I was able to take my baby out in a pram. I was so, so grateful for her. I was also grateful for all my experiences around pregnancy which have been of great use in helping support clients with fertility issues. As is to be expected, I experienced some blood sugar and hormonal upsets, sleep deprivation and the anxieties of a first time Mum, but I didn't suffer from postnatal depression.

However, two years later, just after my granny died, I began to experience anxiety attacks and succumbed to a virulent virus that lasted for weeks. Was I going to fall back into ME again? I recovered, and we all breathed a sigh of relief, but there was yet another hurdle to come.

In 2016 I did a lot of work on myself. I went on a meditation retreat and took an energy course - to better understand myself and the role of the ego in my life. I also experienced a 'healing chamber' which tends to uncover 'stuff' from the subconscious. For me, this revealed a fear of losing those I love and it coincided with Sophia starting school. While I was excited for her and felt fine about it, below the surface, unresolved issues were at work.

My external life was great. I had a partner, a job, and a beautiful child starting school. Why was my internal world suddenly going crazy? Paralysing anxiety was debilitating me to such an extent that coping with day to day life became almost impossible. Some days I couldn't even manage to load the washing machine, or cook dinner. I had never experienced such overwhelming emotions. Fear coursed through my body. Thoughts raced through my mind at an incredible speed. Panic, anger, despair, anxiety and insomnia became so overwhelming that I could hardly get out of bed. So crushing that I did not want to be here. I felt so horrible inside that I began to hit myself and even jagged a knife into my stomach once (luckily I was wearing sturdy jeans at the time). I believed I was losing my mind. I was having a mental breakdown. People must wonder how it's possible to feel this way with a lovely daughter a loving husband and inspiring work, but life isn't that simple.

Terrified that I would never feel well again, would never enjoy my life, my family, my daughter or my work again, I desperately wanted to be fixed! I was ready to try anything and my GP prescribed medication. When I had had ME, they gave me antidepressants, and I had experienced suicidal thoughts. I was desperate enough to take the risk, but they simply sent me to an even darker place. Not to say that they can't help others move forward, but this wasn`t what happened in my case.

> Sometimes when my mind was whizzing
> thoughts flying through my head,
> I wanted to run, escape, switch off
> and cuddle down in bed!

Although I knew that alcohol acts as a depressant and messes with the chemicals in your brain, I was desperate for something to damp down my feelings - to make the bad feelings go away. Of course with alcohol, like drugs, you need more and more to produce an initial feeling of relaxation. After drinking most days for nearly a year, it wasn't until I finally reached rock bottom that something clicked. I went to see an alcohol counsellor and energy therapist called Zoe. She recommended exercise as way to cope with my raging emotions.

Disciplining myself to go to the gym every day was a struggle, but I persevered because exercise burns off the stress hormones produced by fear and anxiety, as well as boosting the happy chemicals in the brain. In the beginning, my thoughts were just as fast and busy, but after I while, I forced myself to visualise pictures of rainbows, peace doves, love hearts, and flowers – to focus on something pleasant and I began my path back to recovery.

It's important to note here that every bout of physical or mental illness I experienced, although difficult and challenging, assisted me to grow. My first illness led to my becoming a nutritionist, and my nervous breakdown empowered me to help others by passing on the simple methods that guided me back to health. I now have a much more rounded view of what constitutes a healthy lifestyle, and the following chapters will explain the tools that helped me find inner peace and wellbeing:

- Friends and family (intimate relationships)
- Monitoring and changing thought patterns
- Practicing relaxation
- Taking exercise
- Letting go (going with the flow)
- Getting to know who you are as an individual (what makes you tick)
- Setting intentions / Using affirmations
- Learning to love yourself / Self-compassion
- Practising gratitude
- Slowing down
- Understanding energy / Spiritual awakening
- Parenting tools (how to cope with being a Mum)
- Good nutrition and creating healthy but tasty recipes

For all of you who have suffered physical or mental illness, I fervently hope that my journey and the tools I used and continue to use to maintain a healthy, balanced lifestyle, will help you at whatever stage you are along your path. Even if you are familiar with many of these concepts, even a phrase that resonates (when the time is right) can help kick-start you on the way from stressed to blessed.

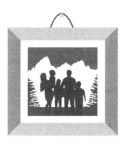

Chapter Two

RELATIONSHIPS AND SUPPORT

You can feel so alone at times
with such difficult feelings inside.
Believe you me there are people who care
so please don't try and hide.

BEING anxiety-ridden, depressed, ill or low in mood is bound to affect relationships. My poor husband John was an unwavering witness to negativity, tears, tantrums, and fears. Yet, I remember him saying almost despairingly "I just want my wife back." Sophia also knew her Mummy wasn't herself because of course children pick up on whatever is going on around them.

Even though I knew my family and friends loved me, I felt that there was no way they could understand what was going on. I felt unworthy, that I was letting everyone down. Even though it felt incredibly lonely, I withdrew from seeing friends because I didn't want to go out socially, fearing that people wouldn't like me if they knew what was going on inside. So my world became smaller and smaller.

Nevertheless, my family persevered. They kept telling me how much they loved me. They helped distract me from negative thoughts by taking me out for a walk, for a cup of tea, or to the garden centre. My parents even had me to stay for a few weeks to take the pressure off household tasks and help take care of Sophia. When I felt I was going crazy and didn't want to be alone, family members made sure I had someone to sit and talk to - someone to whom I could express my fears.

Feeling down, stressed, or ill, messes up the beneficial brain chemicals, which in turn affects your perceptions of yourself. Having faith and hope in yourself and your future when you are caught up in negative thoughts and feelings seems impossible. Being able to speak to professionals over the telephone was a service that helped. www.sane.org.uk has a helpline offering confidential emotional support, as well as calming, downloadable recordings and a wealth of other resources. http://www.supportline.org.uk is another mine of information which also has a helpline. Two other useful resources for anyone suffering from any form of anxiety include www.anxietyuk.org.uk and www.mind.org.uk.

Putting a plan into place encompassing a mix of family, friends, and professionals provided me with a secure platform from which to move forward. It built trust, shone light on my darkness, and helped me gain insight into who I am. We all need support and compassion, and asking for help is a sign of strength. 'No man is an island' and having people tell me that I could and would recover, began to make a difference. I started to open up. Colleagues at the café where I worked part-time were surprisingly non-judgemental encouraging me to view this period as a phase that would pass. I made a friend of another parent at my daughter's Tae Kwon Do class who had experienced anxiety in the past and who let me talk about how I felt, offering support whenever I might need it. And when I finally opened up to my dad, he gave me the biggest hug. I don't think I had had a cuddle like that from him since I was a little girl!

I would never have got this far without the help of family, friends, doctors, and the healing practitioners who gave me acupuncture, reiki, hypnotherapy, and counselling. I am everlastingly grateful to the people who accepted me when I felt so alone. So please don't be alone, open up and talk to someone - whoever that is for you.

Although I still experience some anxiety and low moods from time to time (usually when I have too much on my plate and feel overwhelmed, or comparing myself to others, or not feeling good enough), I know how to help myself. Being honest, knowing what I can manage, and what are the priorities, I gently tell myself to focus on one thing at a time - hard with a fast and furious mind!

Gaining an understanding of ourselves leads towards nourishing and supporting ourselves physically, emotionally and spiritually. Listening to our inner selves leads to self-empowerment, and once we have raised our spirits enough, we can begin to look at putting together a life that suits us, and that works for us in a healthy and balanced way.

> There is a voice inside of you
> that whispers all day long,
> "I feel that this is right for me,
> I know that this is wrong."
> No teacher, preacher, parent, friend
> or wise man can decide
> what's right for you –
> just listen to the voice
> that speaks inside.
> *Sherstein*

Chapter Three

THE MIND AND OUR THOUGHTS

AS well as the marked increase in physical health issues over the last few decades, there has been a rise in mental health and brain disorders. I suggest that it is due in part to a 24/7 lifestyle. We are overwhelmed with information, technology, work, family, and pressure from a society that is trying to dictate how we should live our lives.

The way we think and react is due to a combination of genetics, personality, experiences and conditioning and can also depend on how we are feeling. If we are stressed, or suffering from low blood sugar, or a debilitating virus, our thoughts and reactions can become severely distorted.

On average we think between 60-80,000 thoughts per day – most of them negative and recurring! Mind chatter and overthinking are not only irksome but also cause loss of energy. I should know as I am an over thinker! It is crystal clear that when we are constantly thinking and analysing, we don't enjoy life as much. By changing our inner thoughts our external world improves. When we become aware of our negative thoughts, we can acknowledge them, accept them and change them. It takes work, but it is so worth it because it transforms our lives.

Many therapies are available to help make those changes. Cognitive Behavioural Therapy is extremely valuable in this respect. It teaches that anxiety is an imagined danger which triggers feelings and sensations in the body which cause fight and flight hormones to kick in when they are not needed. These hormones cause us to be hyper-vigilant and even more anxious, exaggerating dangers and underestimating our ability to cope.

One of the best things I have learnt over the years is that what our mind tells us is often untrue. "I am a failure." "No-one is ever going to love me." "I'll never get better." Are these familiar refrains? We can't take everything the mind says seriously! Here are some insights which may be of help:

- Take the focus away from your thoughts and fears by engaging in something you like doing: solving puzzles, cooking something delicious, watching a TV programme.
- Try putting any thoughts you don't like in your SPAM box!
- Challenge your thoughts: Are you really a bad person? Is it true that you will never feel well again, what is the evidence?
- Write down negative thoughts and worries to get them out of your head.
- Focus on what you want, not on what you don't want.
- As you become more aware of negative thoughts, try not to let them build. Stop. Address them and move them in a more positive direction.
- Try to refocus by thinking of a lovely place, or someone you love.
- Look at the sky or flowers.
- Remember fun times.
- Remember things you have achieved.
- See your thoughts printed on clouds and watch them float away.
- Thoughts come and go, ebb and flow. Let them be, just observe them. This is the nature of being human.

I have also learnt that outside influences don't control how I feel. My reactions to what people are saying, or what I think they are saying or even thinking, are inside my head! So my reactions and thoughts about that situation are entirely my responsibility and therefore it is within my control to react positively and move away from negativity which may not even be there! Thoughts and feelings, beliefs and emotions physically change our biochemistry. Negative thoughts and feelings release stress chemicals, while positive, warm and uplifting thoughts and feelings produce beneficial chemicals. Focusing our thoughts on our fears generates more fear, while focusing on peaceful ideas makes us feel peaceful. Leaving anxious thoughts alone, allows the anxiety to subside on its own! Anxiety is covering up the peace we already possess deep inside. While our emotional mind dwells on distressing thoughts and feelings, we also possess a wise mind that is our inner knowing and intuition. We can tap into that wise mind at any time and think about love, beauty, peace, nature and the people we love, which positively affects not only ourselves but those around us. When we start to think better thoughts, we begin to feel better inside. And when we feel a little better, it's good to let pleasant thoughts and sensations drift away because good feelings return more quickly if we don't try to hold onto them! I am learning that outside influences don't control how I feel, it is my thoughts about them, and that realisation can help me to move on. I can have a thought about not being good enough, or successful enough, or pretty enough or whatever but that is only a thought, it is not who I truly am – which at a deep level is a kind and loving human being.

"It is a revelation that we are not our thoughts in our head or our Ego voice - we are the one who sees this." *Eckhart Tolle*

It takes time to change automatic thoughts and reactions. After periods of calm, I'd find that my worrisome mind chatter would start up again and I'd feel disappointed and want to give up! I persevered because I understood that calming my mind by retraining the brain would bring me back to normality.

Spending even a few minutes in meditation can restore calm and inner peace. It's simple, it's inexpensive, and it doesn't require any equipment and has been practised for thousands of years. Meditation benefits both emotional well-being and overall health. It can also help stabilise blood sugar, reduce inflammation and boost energy to name a few benefits. There are classes to join, meditation apps to download, and an array of different types of meditations available on YouTube, including loving kindness meditations. As the Dalai Lama says "wishing others well increases our own happiness. "

Mindfulness is growing worldwide. Mindfulness allows us to see our thoughts and feelings pass through our awareness without judgement - not trying to change them, or fight them, or wish they were different. Mindfulness also teaches us to enjoy pleasant feelings without trying to hold onto them. Our thoughts and feelings are always changing – just like the weather in Scotland!

Try to let your thoughts and feelings
gently flow on by
Try to focus on external beauty
like the trees, flowers and sky.

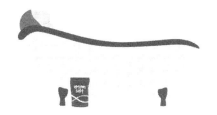

Chapter Four

RELAXATION AND STRESS REDUCTION

Breathing deeply and slowly
calms both body and mind.
Doing this quite regularly
helps in many ways, I find!

TENSION is the body's natural response to stress and worry. Relaxation and breathing techniques help relieve tension. Relaxation and deep breathing help us to feel energised, focused, happier, release heavy feelings, and help us to sleep better. Deeper, slower, rhythmical breathing brings more air into our lungs, relaxing the body and mind which helps us to feel calmer. Many of us tend to hold our breath or breathe more quickly when feeling stressed, rushed, or under pressure. I find that stopping for a minute or two to breathe slowly and rhythmically makes me a feel a lot better before I continue my day.

> "As long as you are breathing, there is more right with you
> than wrong with you!"
> Dr John Kabatzium

When we physically relax our body, the mind automatically follows. Here are some suggestions which have helped me:

- Spend a few minutes each day consciously deep breathing to calm both mind and body.
- Breathing in for 4, holding for 7 and exhaling for 8, can help reduce anxiety. (Exhaling a longer out breath tell us we are safe and that there is no danger).
- Place your hands on your abdomen and watch the rise and fall when you breathe - this simple technique helps to calm a racing mind.
- While breathing try:
  - breathing in calmness and breathing out tension
  - breathing in confidence and breathing out fears and worries
  - say to yourself "I am releasing tension from my mind and body."
  - As you breathe repeat positive words in your mind such as "peace" or "love".
  - Putting your hand over your heart helps calm body and mind (try visualising someone you love at the same time)
  - Find mantras that resonate with you such as "I am doing well," or "I don't have to be perfect."
  - Gently come back to the breath throughout the day

Spending time in silence away from noise, digital and sensory overload helps us to rebalance. Try sitting on a chair with your feet firmly on the floor. Close your eyes. Take some slow deep breaths. Feel strong in your body - like a mountain. Visualise yourself in a safe place – on a beach, in a beautiful garden, in your granny's kitchen – and let thoughts or feelings wash over you.

There are phone apps to help with all these techniques. YouTube offers many resources from binaural beats for anxiety and depression to every kind of mantra.

Music is another great tool. In 2011 a British band joined forces with a group of sound therapists to create the most relaxing tunes ever – you can find them at http://www.makeuseof.com/tag/most-relaxing-songs-all-time-science. And why not try dancing and jigging around the room to your favourite bands. It can't help but lift your spirits!

Listening to music can help to lift your mood and soul.
It helps you feel calmer and happier!
Try it – it just may help you out of a hole.

- After a busy day try putting your legs up a wall for a few minutes. It helps calm and relax the nervous system and improves the levels of energy and oxygen to the head.
- Epsom salt baths remove toxins and aid relaxation and sleep. Put 2-3 cups in a warm bath and soak for 20-30 minutes to release negative emotions.
- Stepping away from computers and phones for about an hour before bed helps promote better sleep. I like listening to relaxing music and reading a book instead (nothing heavy though).
- Spending time in nature can also be tremendously calming. Walking barefoot in the grass or on the beach helps us to ground which makes us feel stronger as well as calmer.
- And let us not forget laughter! It can lighten a mood, release tension, boost our immunity, increase blood flow, and can help us to age better.

- Watching funny clips on YouTube and funny movies also help.
- As does being silly with your children; dressing up; making up silly stories and poems, and bouncing on a trampoline.

> As adults, we can often be
> too serious, busy and stressed.
> Take some time to dance and have fun.
> It can help us feel more blessed!

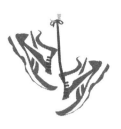

Chapter Five

EXERCISE

OUR bodies are made to move. Scientists have concluded that one of the best ways to beat fatigue and boost energy is to exercise more, not less. Exercise can improve energy levels by strengthening the circulation and heart muscle. New research indicates that sitting is the new smoking, so standing has also become important!

To burn off the excess adrenalin I was generating through stress, and break up the endless cycle of negative thoughts created by my anxiety; I was told that I needed to exercise more, that my daily walk just wasn't enough. So, despite a great deal of resistance on my part, exercise suddenly became a core part of my day, before work, after work, or when Sophia was at school.

When I first started at the gym, my thoughts were fast and busy, but as I said before, I tried to vary them by imagining pictures of rainbows, peace doves, love hearts, and flowers. I also worked on fixing my attention on my body, which shifted my thinking away from negative thoughts.

As my mood improved, I began to notice that I had more energy, and a greater ability to carry out everyday tasks. The exercise was helping me to breathe more deeply and taking in more oxygen was sharpening my brain and elevating my mood! Going to the gym also meant that I was able to spend time with my sister, and however bad I was feeling inside, a little chat with her always helped lift my spirits. After a while, I challenged myself to smile and talk to people I didn't know. Making conversation with people at the gym continues to lift my spirits, and helps me feel connected to other people.

Any movement can help us change how we feel. Doing star jumps in the kitchen, stretching when we get out of bed, dancing, doing a few yoga poses, getting up from the desk away from the computer every 20 minutes to move and stretch, and even doing housework can help us feel energised, sharpen our thinking, and reduce tension. Some of the benefits of regular exercise include:

- Helping to balance weight
- Helping with co-ordination
- Supporting heart health
- Supporting detoxification
- Supporting joints and posture
- Supporting good blood pressure, blood sugar and cholesterol levels
- Strengthening the immune system
- Delivering oxygen and nutrients to cells in our body
- Improving muscle strength
- Improving energy levels
- Helping with pain management
- Helping to release frustration and stress
- Promoting better sleep, memory and concentration
- Stimulating brain chemicals such as endorphins and serotonin which help us to feel happier and more relaxed
- Encouraging positive thoughts

- Boosting confidence and self-esteem
- Social connection

Exercising outside in the fresh air offers even more benefits:

- Aids digestion (it's good to take a walk after a meal)
- The increased oxygen intake delivers even more serotonin, leaving you more refreshed and relaxed
- Cleanses your lungs and sharpens your brain
- Elevates your immune system because white blood cells require a supply of oxygen to fight germs and bacteria

Exercise has become part of my daily life. I go to the gym several times a week, jog or walk outside, or do a little yoga and swim. I really appreciate my body - it allows me to move and exercise! Appreciating it also takes the focus away from the parts that I don't like so much!

In summary, exercise has played a major part in helping me get better. Always check with your GP before starting an exercise programme, especially if you have any medical condition.

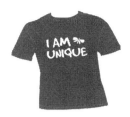

Chapter Six

BEING AN INDIVIDUAL

EACH of us is unique. Each one of us has different skills, abilities, characteristics and experiences. All of us have achieved something whether it be having a family, gaining a qualification, finding work, doing volunteer work, or travelling. And we all do these things differently because we are all different.

So, how do we want to spend our time? Most of us have commitments we need to fulfil each day, but if I have half-an-hour to spare, do I want to spend it doing the housework, or would I rather read a book or do some colouring-in? Life is not always about what we think we 'should' do but what we would like to do. It is important to take the time to engage in activities that bring us joy. What do we love doing? We need to discover what makes us feel good, or calm, or happy. When we put ourselves under pressure, we then need to rebalance. We might want to rest, have fun, or connect with others. Here are some things I have learnt about myself as an individual:

- I need a routine (not too rigid!)
- I need social contact but also need time to myself - to breathe, to rest, or listen to music
- I feel happiest when I feel calm and present

- I feel at my best when I have exercised and eaten well
- I love Epsom salt baths
- I love reading in bed
- I love passing on the information I have learnt to help others
- I love cuddling and having fun with Sophia
- I love rock climbing and ice skating with Sophia
- I love swinging on swings at the park
- I love spending time in the fresh air admiring different landscapes - whatever the weather
- I enjoy writing my Facebook nutrition posts
- I enjoy a good film, a cup of tea with a friend, and a chat at the school drop off
- I enjoy massage and reflexology
- I enjoy activities that don't require thinking - growing veg, cooking new recipes and colouring-in!
- I like slowing down (I tend to rush which makes me feel frazzled)
- I like spending a little time each day just being - looking out of the window at the sky or trees
- I also need a purpose:
    - being the best Mum I can be to Sophia
    - helping others through my work as a nutritionist
    - volunteering at Sophia's school
    - being compassionate to others in my daily life

When I asked Sophia what she thought her Mummy could offer the world I thought she might say helping kids and adults with their nutrition, but she said kindness!

There are many self-help books, blogs and webinars to help us discover ourselves. Ideas, teachings and authors will resonate with us at different times in our lives but the key is to act on what we learn, be it slowing down, exercising, eating better or meditating!

Take time out to relax, recharge
or just sit and simply be,
What is it that can help you?
A bath, music, yoga or a cup of tea?

Chapter Seven

ACCEPTING, LETTING GO AND LETTING FLOW

WISHING I was further along on my healing journey caused me so much anxiety. It took me ages to understand the importance of acceptance, that it was vital to accept how I felt on any particular day. Constantly wishing I was feeling better, calmer and less anxious was counterproductive. The Supremes sing about how "you can`t hurry love!" Nor can you hurry healing or recovery.

Accepting doesn't mean giving up – it just means acknowledging how we feel in the present moment. However much we may want things to be different from how they are in the moment, that burning desire only causes more stress and pain. I think this is one of the hardest things I had to acknowledge. I thought if I read this book, or go to that workshop it would fix me. Not possible! It took me a while to grasp and learn that introducing a mix and match of exercise, good nutrition, positive thinking, relaxation, social connection and fun little by little, would result in a balanced life.

Here are some examples of things I stopped fighting and learnt to accept – because resisting caused them to persist. Fighting a particular feeling blocks the possibility of flowing into a different feeling!

- I have sensations of anxiety in my chest; I don't like it!

  Accept, breathe and let go.

- If I let myself feel angry what might happen?

  Not judging allows a different feeling in, be it happy or sad.

- Being a mum is wonderful and tiring!

  That is how it is! Accept it

- The house is often untidy.

  Of course, it is. I have a child! Accept it.

- Young children often interrupt you, demand your attention and have tantrums!

  It's natural. It's what they do.

- A client cancelled. My day isn't going to plan!

  It's not the end of the world. It's okay.

- I react very strongly to noise, energy, and food.

  Okay, I have a super sensitive system and need to learn to manage it.

- Sophia is growing up, and I am getting older.

  That's as it should be. I'm not 20 and don't gad about town anymore. I have a different life now.

- The weather in Scotland is changeable.

  We can't always plan outdoor activities – but there are other things we can do.

- Every day is different. How I feel. What I do.

  I won't try to hold on to how I was yesterday. I accept that sometimes I feel happy and calm, and sometimes anxious, sad or tense.

- I keep repeating the same mistake.

  I accept my weakness without judgement - but will do better next time.

○ Everyone is different in the way they think and react. It is futile to hope that others will change or mould themselves into how I want them to be.

I accept that my husband John was never going to wear designer clothes, dance on tables, or drive a motorbike!

○ Good feelings come and go. As humans, we ebb and flow through many feelings in the course of a day.

I will savour the good moments and the good feelings in my body.

Thoughts and feelings aren't permanent. They are able to flow through the body and be released. I often ask my anxiety, excess adrenalin, tension or heaviness to flow down to my feet and out into the earth. Most of the time it works, but like anything, practice makes perfect. Incidentally, both caffeine and sugar trigger the stress hormone adrenalin.

I quite like the word 'charge' instead of stress. It feels lighter. If Sophia is playing up or irritating me, I ask the 'charge' of Sophia to flow through me and visualise a white light helping the frustration flush away. Then Sophia often says "Let the charge of Mummy flow through me" which makes us both laugh!

Sometimes I whisper "soften the tension" or "let this irritation flow through me" and immediately feel a difference! There was time when I used to scream and shout about how I hated my thoughts and feelings. Now I can observe, acknowledge and even turn them around. At the very least I can change focus because "…what we focus on grows".

Working with an energy therapist or counsellor helped me understand my thoughts and feelings and set me on the path of letting them go.

Emotions and moods can come and go
We start to understand this the more we learn and grow,
Nothing stays the same so instead of hanging on
Let thoughts and feelings pass through and flow

We sometimes feel balanced
Sometimes up and down
Sometimes we have a natural smile
At other times we scowl and frown!

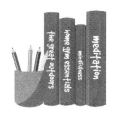

Chapter Eight

AFFIRMATIONS AND INTENTIONS

AFFIRMATIONS are phrases designed to affect the mind positively - to motivate, energise, calm, or keep us focused. They help put us in a better frame of mind and so feel better inside. They are not a magic cure but at the very least another tool to help us move away from focusing on what we think is wrong with us.

Repeating affirmations made a real difference if I repeated them when I felt overwhelmed or anxious. I also found that writing affirmations in a notebook at the same time each day was also extremely helpful. Here are some of my favourites:

- ○ This too shall pass
- ○ I will come out of this
- ○ All is well in this moment
- ○ I am enough
- ○ I am worthy of love, peace and joy
- ○ I am growing and learning so much
- ○ I am calm and strong - I can cope
- ○ I am healthy and full of energy
- ○ I am safe now

- I am filled with light and love
- One moment, one breath
- One day at a time, one step at a time
- I go with the flow of life

Another useful antidote to dark times is to write down wishes and desires. Here are some of mine:

- Being more present
- Inner peace and calm
- Feeling lighter about life
- Helping others with work that I enjoy
- Running workshops
- Meetings with family and friends
- More fun
- More travel
- More short breaks

Sometimes I add gratitude for feelings or events - as if they had already happened and suddenly I find that I am feeling those feelings:

- Thank you for a bit of fun today
- Thank you for feelings of peace
- Thank you for helping me make connections with others
- Thank you for helping me cope with the day well
- I also make lists of things I want to let go of:
  - Feeling stressed
  - Overthinking
  - Self-criticism

I regularly ask Angels for help. I often ask for love and light to fill me up both for myself and those I meet. Turning to a Higher Power for help in whatever form is simple and direct. Affirmations help too, I was attracted to this affirmation in a magazine and often repeat it before I go to sleep: "The more I go with life, the better my life will be. I expect the Universe to send me what I need. I work through my fears. My career is expanding"!

Chapter Nine

SELF-LOVE AND SELF-COMPASSION

Treat yourself wonderfully well.
You deserve the very best.
This to yourself be sure to tell!

ACCEPTANCE, self-love and self-compassion are vital keys to our long-term happiness.

I spent years comparing myself to others both personally and professionally, feeling that I wasn't good enough. How come I was able to recognise positive qualities, skills and talents in others, but unable to validate my own? Constant self-comparison to others on Facebook, at work, or even to strangers on the street can knock our self-esteem and bring us down. Comparing ourselves to others is futile, and we have no idea what their lives are really like or what they are feeling on the inside! Did you know that self-criticism triggers the release of stress hormones in the body?

By simply becoming aware of this trait is a major step to changing the way we view ourselves. Then, by focusing on our positive characteristics, we can begin to change our opinion of ourselves for the better, lighten our mood, feel better inside, and have more energy.

The beauty of you lies inside.
Temporarily covered up.
There's light and love and laughter there.
A beautiful flowing cup.

Juggling modern life is hard, and there is so much pressure on us all to 'succeed'. A successful life looks and feels different for each of us. Practising self-love and self-compassion helps balance mind and body which creates a firm foundation on which to build a successful life. So here are some ideas around self-love. Kindness to oneself can include:

- Making a list of what we appreciate about ourselves
- Accepting how we are right now (which doesn't mean not wanting to move forward in various areas)
- Remembering we don't have to be perfect!
- Repeating the mantra "I am enough just as I am"
- Using kind self-talk instead of chastising ourselves with harsh words
- Feeding ourselves well
- Taking time out
- Taking part in activities we enjoy
- When in the midst of anxiety, fear or depression, giving ourselves a pat on back for small achievements such as
  - doing the dishes
  - making dinner
  - getting your child to school
  - getting out and going for a walk
- Listing the day's successes, however small, before going to sleep

- Raising our self-worth by showing kindness to others in simple ways such as offering a smile and a kind word to strangers at a bus stop or
- Saying no!

Another way of showing compassion to ourselves when we are struggling and perhaps feeling sorry for ourselves is by comforting ourselves physically! Stroking a body part such as an arm or a leg produces calming chemicals and relaxes the brain. Thanks Angie Cameron for this awareness!

An unexpected benefit of appreciating and loving ourselves more is that sugar and junk food become less important. Changing our relationship with food also changes our relationship with ourselves. When we eat well, we feel more nourished and exercise becomes easier, as does putting ourselves first. An important factor I noticed while I was practising these changes was that when I congratulated myself on mastering a particular negative behaviour, I was more aware when the behaviour returned! It was a little less intense and lasted for a shorter time. The process of retraining ourselves to be kind and compassionate to ourselves takes time, and effort but is so worth it!

Be compassionate with yourself.
Take baby steps onward.
By trusting your own wise self,
you move gently forward.

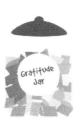

Chapter Ten

GRATITUDE

GRATITUDE reduces sadness and fear and helps us feel happier. Gratitude helps us focus on the good in our lives, however small.

Gratitude helped me take the focus off what I thought was wrong with me, my health and my life. The more I practised gratitude, the better I felt. Thinking about what we haven't yet achieved - more friends, better work, more money, or better health makes us feel unhappy. Shifting focus by concentrating on the friends, work, money and good health that we do have, attracts more of the same! Here are some suggestions to start building awareness of what is good in your life:

- At the end of the day write down one or two things that you are grateful for and put them in a jar labelled 'my gratitude jar'!
- Before going to sleep say out loud, or write in a notebook, five things you have been grateful for during the day
- Try being grateful for the present moment
- Be grateful for what you have already learnt and achieved
- Several times a day stop and focus on something to be grateful for - noticing and appreciating the small things

If you are on a healing or learning journey, try to notice small improvements instead of focusing on what is still 'wrong', or still needs work. Try gratitude for being in the presence of something larger than yourself - you might be in awe of nature, the sky, witnessing random acts of kindness

Some of the things I have been grateful for and have said thank you for:

- My family, daughter, friends, lovely people I know
- What my body does for me daily without my even asking it: circulating blood, digesting food, moving, seeing
- Therapists who have supported me on my journey
- The view out of my window – a garden with trees and flowers
- The feel of Sophia's soft skin
- The lovely colours, pictures and love hearts in my house
- A warm bath or shower
- My clients
- Interactions at the gym and café
- Sharing with a friend over a cup of tea
- When my husband John cooks me a meal
- Friends who have not judged me in my darkest moments
- Watching Sophia and her friends playing
- Watching TV with my family
- Progress I have made
- Lightness and moments of calm - if only for a few seconds
- My gran leaving me a little money which led to a family holiday
- My eyes revealing the beauty all around: sky, flowers, birds, sea

When we respond to something we find beautiful, it alters the pattern of our brainwaves. Beautiful moments bring joy, calm the nervous system and lessen our stress response, enabling us to lift our mood, feel happy, relax and recharge. Beauty and simple pleasures are all around us. We simply need to deliberately look for beauty in the day – smells, colours, sounds, fun. Can't find anything? Look for beautiful memories! Here are some of mine:

- Seeing a rainbow in the sky, looking at flowers, hearing the birds sing
- Looking at Sophia's face
- Colouring-in, or doing sticker books with Sophia
- Lying on the grass watching clouds float by for a few seconds before Sophia and her friend jumped on me!
- Running round trees with Sophia
- Listening to children laughing
- Watching children's TV with Sophia - Octonauts, Postman Pat, Paw Patrol – so funny and with great animation!
- Spontaneous laughter – laughter improves mood and bodily functions
- Being the silly version of myself with friends - nice to feel less serious about life even if only for a few moments
- The sheer warmth and happiness from a group hug with kids in the classroom where I volunteer
- Connecting with children as I help them with their writing work
- Bopping to music in the car after a mindfulness meditation which helped release tension and tightness in my chest
- Dancing with Sophia in the kitchen
- When Sophia said "I love you" out of the blue - without wanting something!
- Saying goodnight to angels, birds, flowers, trees at the window with Sophia

○ Cuddling Sophia in the morning with a cup of green tea

○ Listening to music with eyes closed

○ A weekend away with the family without internet connection – we were all so much more present, and I saw my parents not just as parents but as people!

○ Going for a jog around Pittencrieff Park and sitting in the beautiful walled gardens for a wee while

○ Walking with Sophia and other fairies in the Galaday

It seems that modern life demands us to think and act big, that bigger is better. What about the small and beautiful? Small things can make a big impact - a smile, a compliment, a kind word or gesture; having a cuddle; a small gap in the day to rest, making a small portion of healthy food; or simply looking out of the window at a flower or a bird.

> "Be happy with what you have,
> while working for what you want..."
> *Helen Keller*

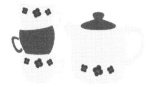

Chapter Eleven

WHAT'S THE RUSH? BECOMING MORE PRESENT

RUSHING, multi-tasking and feeling hurried increases the stress fight or flight response. Over time, it can even cause negative emotional and physical symptoms. Training our body and mind to slow down helps release us from being in stress mode all the time. I always seemed to be rushing. My mind always one step ahead thinking about the next thing to do or achieve. I even read the last few pages of a book to see what was going to happen! Such impatience! Why? Genetics, hardwiring, upbringing? Women's brains are programmed to multi-task, to think ahead, and assess what needs to be accomplished. Some people appear to thrive this way, but I find multi-tasking both stressful and exhausting! For me, completing one task after another just isn't living. If I catch myself rushing to get out the door - especially on school drops offs – I stop, take a breath and re-calibrate! I finally understood that the rushing was all in my mind.

Dr David Hamilton, who uses science to inspire, suggests: "Our sense of the need to hurry makes things harder. Choosing not to rush and take less action can make things easier and certainly feels nicer inside." www.drdavidhamilton.com

Instead of pushing and striving to achieve all the time, I try to listen to what my body needs. I try to be present in a task, complete it, and then take a break with a cup of tea before moving on to the next activity. Just taking that short break gets me off the treadmill of constantly doing. Slowing down helps us feel more joyful. While it takes time to programme our brains and minds to focus solely on the task at hand, it can be done. Young children are more naturally in the present moment - we could take a leaf out of their book!

> Young children can be so focused
> on the activities they do
> they can become so absorbed
> that when you speak
> you think they are ignoring you!

As we get caught up in the business of life, try remembering that each day and each moment is special - without thinking ahead. When we bring our attention to the present, we take our thoughts away from the past, or future. We realise that life is happening right now, in this moment, whatever it may be. Cooking, doing the dishes, doing homework with the children, a work project, exercising, or doing housework. Being present eases stress, gives more joy and can help us feel more connected to life.

While it is good to have goals, day-to-day life is not all about doing and achieving, but also about acts of kindness, compassion, and loving. And it isn't always about the result; enjoyment is also found in the process. I have often missed out on enjoying something because I have been impatient to get it finished. Of course being in the moment doesn't mean we can't plan or put structure in place – but it's better to plan when not trying to iron or cook at the same time! Here are some of my tips on slowing down:

○ Try taking on fewer tasks each day.

○ Create some down time.

○ Watch your sense of urgency to get things done (this is a biggy for me).

○ Give yourself a pat on the back on completion of a task before rushing on to the next.

○ Write down in your diary or planner what you want to achieve that day - be honest about how realistic that is and try to keep to it. A day for me might involve taking Sophia to school, going to the gym, seeing clients, a little clearing up in the house, and preparing a meal.

○ Try to set a time limit for a task and stick to it. I used to go on and on and on and tire myself out!

○ Doing one thing at a time helps conserve energy and wellbeing.

○ When you feel yourself agitated, rushing or revving up, pause, breathe, and look out the window, or at something beautiful.

○ Although it's fine to think of lovely places, it's better to enjoy the here and now! (When it's raining in Scotland, I sometimes wish I was on a beach in Spain or Australia.)

○ Becoming aware of sounds, sights, smells, helps to be 'in the moment'! I often concentrate on the shapes and details in pictures and photos.

○ When I am playing with Sophia, instead of thinking about what I need to do next, I focus on the softness of Sophia's skin or the beauty of her eyes.

○ Acknowledging the moments or minutes when we feel good, calls in more of the same.

○ Our butterfly minds have a tendency to wander, so coming back to the present over and over helps to train us to be 'present in the moment'.

○ When I feel present, time seems to expand, and it feels soo much nicer!

Babies, young children and animals live in the moment. They don't think about the future, they are only doing what they are doing. Practising being present can lead to inner peace and happiness. I enjoy my life so much more now that I am working on being present and 'smelling the roses' – not rushing ahead to what's next – although it's still a work in progress.

Being in the present moment
is the very best place to be.
It takes you out of the past or future
Setting your mind totally free.

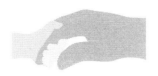

Chapter Twelve

BEING A MUM

BEING a parent is full of highs and lows. It is challenging, demanding, and totally wonderful. No one teaches you how - and it takes a while for the reality to sink in! At the time of writing, my Sophia is six years old - having more strops and attitude than ever before!

We put so much pressure on ourselves to be a perfect parent. We also want our children to be perfect, and when Sophia was younger, I used to compare her progress with that of others, another stressful activity that I stopped. Accepting instead that she was her own little being, doing things in her own time. So what if other children seemed to be walking or talking sooner? Children all progress at their own rate. Each has their own skills, and talents, finding some things easier than others. And we can always turn to our GP or health visitor if there are serious worries.

I found talking to other mums helpful, except when they boasted about their child sleeping through from early on! And I laughed when a friend told me that her husband got so fed up with one of their twins not eating the spaghetti bolognaise that he poured it over his head! I used to get stressed if Sophia wasn't eating too. Not good - babies pick up on our anxiety.

The information I found in books and on the web was helpful, but also full of contradictions. So apart from basic milestones, and 'The Baby

Whisperer' by Tracey Hogg, I stopped reading baby books. Sophia was never going to be a Gina Ford baby! As soon as we got into a routine, it would all change again! I finally learnt to trust my instincts about what was right for her.

Another stressful area involved clearing up the mess that Sophia and her friends continually created, but what was the point of overreacting? I had to let go of that frustration and finally had to accept that mess and children go together!

Children can be beautiful,
loving, honest, mischievous and fun.
They have so much natural energy
to help them skip, scoot and run!

Some of my lessons and observations:

- Time is not our own!
- We are not always in control.
- Sometimes we can't even go to the toilet in peace!
- Children push our buttons and test our patience.
- Children are noisy and make a mess.
- Getting pissed off about constantly tidying up isn't helpful!
- Children need to take responsibility for tidying up.
- Decent adult conversation disappears!
- Embracing the ridiculousness of parenting is helpful!
- Accepting that some days inevitably lead to total exhaustion and a good cry.
- Children follow their own rhythms - sleeping and eating.

- Children push for what they want!
- Children get absorbed in what they are doing and ignore you.
- Children live in the moment.
- Children are bundles of energy and need to be in motion.
- Children are free spirits.
- Children can teach us as the wonder of life.
- Children are all different, and we should allow them to be themselves.
- Children make friends and gain their independence, but they will always need you, love you and come back to you.

Slow down mummy, there is no need to rush,
Slow down mummy, what is all the fuss?
Slow down mummy, make yourself a cup tea.
Slow down mummy, come and spend some time with me.
Slow down mummy, let's put our boots on and go out for a walk,
let's kick at piles of leaves, and smile and laugh and talk.
Slow down mummy, you look ever so tired,
come sit and snuggle under the duvet and rest with me a while.
Slow down mummy, those dirty dishes can wait,
slow down mummy, let's have some fun, let's bake a cake!
Slow down mummy I know you work a lot,
but sometimes mummy, its nice when you just stop.
Sit with us a minute, and listen to our day,
spend a cherished moment,
because our childhood is not here to stay! X

Rebekah Knight www.facebook.com/slowdownmummy

Freedom is so important for children, but so is guidance and discipline. I tend to pick my battles – as when Sophia and her friends scooted out onto the main road path, instead of stopping at the edge of our housing estate! Freedom for Mums and Dads is important too. Recharging batteries and doing what we love to do is important for the ongoing harmony of the home. Whether it's taking a nap, meeting a friend, playing sport, or practising a hobby. We need time to be ourselves - away from caring, washing, cooking and cleaning up. It is vital to look after ourselves well. Eating and sleeping well, enjoying fresh air and exercise is important for the sake of the entire family's well-being.

The whole process of becoming and being a Mum takes its toll on both mind and body. From growing a baby, giving birth, going through hormonal imbalances, experiencing lack of sleep, depleted nutrient reserves, and possibly balancing work and child care. Many Mums lose confidence or experience a kind of post-natal burnout with a feeling of having lost themselves. It can happen right away or up to two years after giving birth. Caught up in the endless round of chores, housework and caring for our child, we can forget our own needs. Parents are not machines! We have to find ways to balance the load so that we can cope with day to day life better, leaving enough energy for the fun side of having kids. The antics of children can make our blood boil, but they can also lift our mood, help us to feel more childlike, and make us smile. Here are some of the joys I have experienced:

○ A warm Scottish spring day. Sophia and her friends were playing pie face, and I put my face through the plastic oval and got creamed! It was funny. It's good to be silly with children now and again.
○ Walking with my primary school children in the Galaday helped me feel such love in my heart.

- One day for no reason Sophia said: "you are the mum of my dreams".
- On a winter's night, Sophia ran out of the house giggling to watch her flashing light slippers twinkle in the dark!
- Dancing to the radio in the kitchen with Sophia and her friends even though I felt shattered. Children can boost your energy as well as drain it!
- Sophia and her friend Hannah were playing hide and seek and asked me to find them. How did I find them under my bed? Sophia had her electric toothbrush on which makes a noise and gave them away!
- Sophia was playing outside with her friends in her swimsuit. It started raining quite heavily, and the next thing I saw was Sophia scooting around the grass in her swimsuit and wellies. We have a photo of her in swimsuit and wellies holding a brolly!
- Painting with Sophia and her friends - their paintings were better than mine!
- Watching TV with Sophia cuddling me and playing with my hair.
- Making fruit kebabs and smoothies and sharing nutrition info with some of the children at Sophia's school.
- Sophia in Granny Bisset's back garden, asking if she could pick some flowers to give to Mummy!
- One day when I was feeling grumpy, I came upon the kids playing air guitar to a radio rock station. They looked so funny; it helped shift my irritation.
- Going down the Helter Skelter, and round the Carousel, I suddenly missed the fun and freedom of being a child.

- One morning before school Sophia said, "I'm setting up a party with balloons and arts and crafts for my toys". Then I heard her shout "Let's get this party started!!" which made me laugh out loud.
- Sometimes, when I've talked about the future, Sophia says "Don't worry about that just yet mummy." Children are so 'present'!
- After watching the Rio Olympics, Sophia started a gymnastic class. When I asked how it was going, she said she was disappointed that she hadn't been allowed to try a cartwheel on the balance beam! Nice to have self-belief!

This amazing little person began a new chapter of joy in my life, and it is an honour and privilege to take care of her.

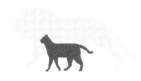

Chapter Thirteen

STARTING TO FEEL BETTER FROM THE INSIDE

If we understand that deep inside
there is sparkle, joy and fun
covered up by fears and thoughts
we unravel to feel the sun

HERE are some more techniques that helped me feel better. Since we are all different, experiment and practice to find the ones that work for you! I often felt helpless when I felt anxious, down, or angry, but thanks to the support of Zoe, Shirley and other therapists, I slowly gained confidence. I began to feel self-empowered and believed that I could change how I felt inside. I made steady but gradual progress by making small positive changes. When it felt too hard, I often felt like giving it up, and although it wasn't helpful, I'd sometimes fly into a rage and shout "well I am f...ing trying" at books and audios! It can be frustrating finding the right tool when thoughts and emotions are crowding in. There's no magic wand, just practice and belief.

- Start to accept where you are and how you are feeling right now. Fighting anxiety symptoms gives them fuel. (We get more of what we focus on.)

○ Feeling your emotions is actually healthy, whereas suppressing, avoiding them or changing them with food, drugs, or alcohol is not.

○ Writing your thoughts and feelings down in a journal gets them out of your head. (I used to write about the fear of never feeling happy or well again.)

○ You can write down how you are feeling and then put an alternative underneath "I feel really anxious" / "I am calm and strong". Then watch the negative thoughts float away.

○ Focus on what you have achieved rather than what you haven't done. Write down even the smallest achievements, small feelings of happiness, acknowledging that the day was not all bad or hard!

○ Praying, meditating, reading, doing puzzles, and colouring-in can calm a racing mind. I even did word searches to try to focus my mind!

○ Thinking of events, people and places that you love can help dispel worrying or negative thoughts and lift you out of a bit of a low.

○ Doing, or thinking about doing what you love, helps dispel the negative chemicals in your body that are triggered by fear, anxiety, anger, worry, etc.

○ If you like visualisation, change a black cloud feeling into a brighter colour; or make it more distant; or see it on a TV screen and then turn off the TV.

○ Screaming or shouting into a pillow or in an appropriate place can help release pent up frustration, irritation and anger. I often say to Sophia "I'm going to roar like a lion." She thinks it's a game and joins in too!

- Any form of exercise can help change negative energy – stretching, dancing, running, or yoga etc. It also increases oxygen to the brain which enables you to make better choices – about the food you eat, how you are dealing with your relationships and life in general.
- Complimenting someone can be so uplifting. I sometimes go deliberately out of my way to be nice to someone and immediately feel happier inside.
- Forcing myself to go out when I didn't feel like it; going to work at my café and speaking to the staff or customers; making myself chat to the other Mums when I took Sophia to a party; or going for a walk rather than putting my head under the duvet, always made me feel a little better.

Becoming more aware of my thoughts, feelings and sensations, like an observer, makes it much easier not to react and to let them pass. "Okay, I have some anxiety feelings in my chest – I'll just accept them for now!" / "I feel a bit low today - that's okay, I know it will pass." That's something I found really hard as I was so fearful of those types of feelings.

I have also taught myself to catch my inner critic - that ego part of ourselves that loves to judge, create dramas, and make mountains out of molehills. When it starts telling me I am not good enough, comparing me to others, or saying that I must do something now, I start laughing kindly, and say: "Oh Anne, there you go again – don't be silly."

Something else I regularly do is sit on the edge of my bed and ask a beautiful white light to come through the crown of my head and fill all my cells with loving, healing light. If you understand the chakra system, you can also ask the white light to fill each chakra up with loving, healing light and to cleanse, clear and rebalance each one. Then take the light down your feet into the earth. I usually do this before bed and feel calmer as a result.

In the morning I sometimes sit quietly and visualise a white light washing away stress, negativity, anxiety and do the same with the water when I am in the shower.

I also like to plant 'seeds' at the beginning of the day by jotting down in my journal how I would like to feel: to have friendly interactions; to feel love inside; experience moments of calmness and happiness. These positive intentions can have a real effect on how we feel overall. I am often surprised at the end of the day when I look back on what I wrote to see how many of my intentions came to pass.

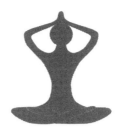

Chapter Fourteen

ENERGY / SPIRITUALITY / AWAKENING

THE food we eat gives us the nutrients to fuel our cells. Exercising increases the oxygen and blood flow around the body. The thoughts we think also affect our flow of energy. There is another type of life force known as chi. Therapies and practices such as reiki, acupuncture, yoga and tai chi can enhance and strengthen this energy, as well as removing tension and blockages improving our overall health.

I am quite sensitive to energies, moods, noise, and the environment. I can feel when someone is upset, and sometimes take on other peoples' anxieties and worries. I have to accept that this is part of me, but I use techniques to help reduce any negative effects by grounding or putting a protective bubble around me. I ask for a protective golden and white light to surround my physical and auric bodies. To let out only good energy from me to others I meet. For any negative or lower energy from others or the environment to be sent out to the universe/nature, etc. and to be dissolved with love!

From the Energy course I did with Zoe, Shirley, and Jacqui, I learnt that we can become sensitive to feeling energy in our hands and feet. When we rub our hands together briskly and feel the energy that generates, it can help us get out of a cycle of fear or anxiety and reduce the stress response the body produces when we feel anxious, stressed or upset. It takes practice, but I have noticed feeling much better when I do stop and do this for a few minutes. It also helps us connect to ourselves.

Another idea, which can take time, is to sit and be with our negative feelings and then watch the energy shift to a different location in the body. But always work with a therapist if you feel this is too much to do on your own.

Negative ions are odourless, invisible molecules that we inhale in natural environments such as beaches, by waterfalls, mountains, forests, rivers. Once they reach our bloodstream, negative ions are believed to produce biochemical reactions that increase levels of our mood chemicals - endorphins and serotonin - helping to reduce depression, relieve stress, calm the nervous system, improve our immunity and boost our daytime energy. I definitely feel calmer and more balanced when I have spent time outside in nature and am lucky to be able to reach beaches, forests, rivers, lochs within an hour from my home.

A few years ago I attended a demonstration of Deeshka which involves a transfer of divine, intelligent energy. The process creates a neurobiological shift in the brain and awakens the chakras in the body. It can produce a shift in consciousness, freeing us from the suffering that is created by the mind. It also helps balance the body's natural energies. Once initiated, this 'awakening' process gradually leads to greater inner peace and wellbeing. Deeshka helps you to connect more directly with the truth of your own being.

What drew me to it initially to was that it helps balance energy from the overactive thinking centres of the brain to the more calming frontal lobes! It assists in rewiring the brain to bring more peace, clarity, feelings of joy, connection to self and others. Feelings and issues that need discarding also come to the surface. Having completed several Deeshka workshops and meditation groups, it has helped open my heart more and I can now give and receive this beautiful, calming energy. It aids the evolution of our planet and does not belong to any religion or belief.

Sometimes big life changes can trigger an 'awakening'. When Sophia was about three years old I woke up in the night and felt as if a lightning bolt was charging through my body. It gave me quite a fright and I didn't know what was happening to me and couldn't get back to sleep. In the morning I was still so befuddled that when I took the car out I forgot to put the handbrake on, and it rolled back into a wall! I now believe that my body was being adjusted to let in more love and light.

I have also read and listened to the spiritual teachings of thought leaders such as Wayne Dyer, Eckhart Tolle, as well as obtaining guidance from my therapists Zoe and Shirley. While these teachings and events mean different things to different people, they do relate to the spiritual side of life but are not about religion. I have written below what 'being spiritual' means to me. Have a wee think about what it means to you.

- Trusting in a higher power - whatever that is
- Learning to let go - not always trying to control outcomes
- Spending more time in nature
- Developing my intuition so that I know what is right for me whether it be the food I am choosing or places to go
- Listening to my inner voice by turning off noise and closing my eyes
- Doing work I enjoy
- Writing and working from the heart to help others
- Thanking the universe and my angels for helping me in my day to day life and helping me to release my fears and anxieties

○ Being grateful for all the good in my life
○ Being kind, compassionate and loving towards myself and others (this is the key element for me)
○ Spending time alone, listening to music, breathing, or meditating
○ Our hearts have their own wisdom and intelligence. Intelligence does not only come from the mind. When we 'think' with our hearts it can enhance our health and wellbeing

With practice, natural shifts take place inside enabling us to feel calmer, more aware and with a clearer understanding of ourselves. Zoe reminds me that we go through cycles in life – a cycle of anxiety, a cycle of flow, and cycles of high and low energy. It is important to understand this as it takes pressure away from always trying to feel great, energised and sorted all the time.

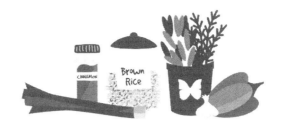

Chapter Fifteen

INTRODUCTION TO NUTRITION

Good nutrition helps our
body, mind and moods
so please eat nourishing meals
with healing, tasty food!

The food we eat is harvested
from earth, land and sea,
providing all the ingredients
for breakfast, lunch and tea!

It gives us many nutrients
which feed organs, bones and skin
protect our eyes, our joints and brain.
You see how beauty comes from within!

Our bodies are fed by
the daily food we eat.
Feed your lifelong vehicle well
and remember to enjoy some treats!

My aim here is to ignite your interest and fan a flame to help you start taking care of you! My passion is to help others understand and believe in the power of food in supporting physical and mental well-being. To start looking at food as a friend to help energise, nourish and keep you well. Our bodies need a healthy balance of nutrients to sustain us, and some of us aren't receiving all the nutrients we need because they are not present in the foods modern society is producing, and particularly in junk and fast food. Please note that I am not writing about specific symptoms or conditions, but offer tips, ideas and interesting nutrition bites which will help support body systems.

What we eat has a great impact on how we feel physically, mentally and emotionally. Food in its natural state supports every part of our body. It not only helps optimize our energy and enthusiasm for life but reduces the risk of disease. It is so important to understand that all the processes that take place in our bodies on a daily basis are to a great extent determined by what we put into our mouths. Our bodies are naturally designed to be well! From keeping bugs at bay and repairing and healing, to digesting food and producing energy. However, modern life appears to be geared to causing dis-ease! New technology, information overload, a media biased toward producing negative news, toxic cleaning products, toxic environmental problems, nutrient poor food, and with people spending less and less time out in the natural world, it is hardly surprising that dis-ease seems to be on the increase. The degree of inflammation in people's bodies is a startling indication of how out of balance we are. Inflammation is a result of poor diet, environmental toxins, stress, and lack of sleep. More and more research links long-term, low-grade inflammation to chronic diseases such as Alzheimer's, cancer, depression, diabetes, and heart disease. So the better quality food you put in, the better your cells and body processes will work, not forgetting the other factors which affect health, including thoughts and emotions, exercise, rest, environment and lifestyle.

What does food mean to you? Energy? Fuel? Medicine? Pleasure? Comfort? Perhaps you view it as a chore? Take a few moments to consider. How about regarding food as the nourishment that helps you feel good on a daily basis throughout your life? Eating well is one of the primary ways of supporting the belief that you matter, that you make a difference in the world, that you are important.

Changing your food and nutrition is a process, it doesn't just happen overnight. Focus on choosing health and well-being instead of thinking about giving up or reducing certain foods, and you will find that eating well begins to feel natural. The more you do it, the easier it gets. When you begin, it can be confusing telling the difference between what our minds are telling us we want to eat, with what our bodies need. The streets are lined with fast food restaurants and supermarket aisles full of processed foods, ready meals, and sugary snacks tempting us to eat products that are nutrient deficient. The stress of a demanding life can trigger cravings for junk food, an addiction to sugar, caffeine and other substances. The good news is that when we are out of balance, symptoms of dis-ease arise like red flags letting us know that there is an issue that needs addressing. Adjusting your diet, getting more fresh air, exercising, and having more fun, go a long way in assisting your healing.

Healthy eating information can be both overwhelming and conflicting, but it is actually very simple: the basis of well-being lies with proper nutrition, and nature provides the food that our bodies are naturally designed to eat.

Everything in this section is the sum of what I have learned as a qualified nutritionist, and what I have personally experienced working through my health issues.

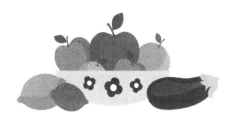

Chapter Sixteen

BASIC CONCEPTS OF NUTRITION

NUTRITION is the study of the food you eat and how your body uses it. We eat food to live, to grow, to keep healthy and well, and to get energy for work and play. It is a foundation of good health.

Food is made up of different nutrients: vitamins, minerals, antioxidants, and essential fats, all of which are absorbed by the body as it passes through the digestive system. Along with fibre, light, oxygen and water, these nutrients are essential for physical and mental health. They take care of cell growth, maintenance, and enable your body to function efficiently. No single food has all the nutrients our bodies require which is why we need to eat a varied and balanced diet for optimal health.

Did you know eating protein at a meal helps feelings of fullness, reduces cravings and keeps your energy more stable?

Did you know that Protein puts the brakes on the brain chemicals that motivate you to reach for food, even when you're not hungry?

Protein
Essential for the body and brain to build new cells for healthy growth and development, tissue growth, and repair of skin and muscles.

- ✓ Meat including beef, lamb, chicken, turkey - free range, grass fed and organic, as your budget allows
- ✓ Fish and shellfish
- ✓ Eggs
- ✓ Dairy products: cow, goat and sheep
- ✓ Beans, lentils, nuts, seeds, tofu and tempeh (soya)
- ✓ Protein powders: whey, hemp, rice, pea - great for adding to smoothies
- ✓ Some vegetables and grains also contain protein - the highest sources are found in sprouted beans, peas and lentils - easy and cheap to sprout yourself!

Carbohydrates

There are two main types of carbohydrates – complex (whole grain), and simple (refined). Whole grain carbohydrates release their sugars more slowly which helps sustain energy levels. Eating too much refined and sugary carbs contributes to weight gain and over time, illness.

Reduce your white and sugary carbs and eat more brown and whole grain varieties:

- ✓ Brown, red and wild rice
- ✓ Oats, quinoa, rice noodles, millet, buckwheat and barley
- ✓ Wholemeal bread, pitta bread, rye bread
- ✓ Whole grain pasta
- ✓ Fruit, veg, beans, and lentils also contain healthy carbs
- ✓ Sweet Potatoes

Did you know sweet potatoes actually support blood sugar levels?

Did you know that Quinoa is a high energy food? It is a grain that is not only gluten free but also high in protein. It was a staple of the Inca people (known for their stamina) and is rich in many nutrients such as B vitamins, magnesium, calcium and iron and supports bone and ligament health.

Fats

Every cell in the body benefits from 'good' fats. The brain and the nervous system are made up of around 60 per cent fat. The right kind of fats keeps the brain and body well oiled. Low-fat diets can lead to depression and anxiety. You need the right kind of fats to boost learning, behaviour and brain development, support your immune system, help your skin glow, protect your eyes, heart and joints, boost your mood and help you lose weight.

The right kind of essential fats are found in:

- ✓ Seeds including pumpkin, coconut, chia, flax, and sunflower
- ✓ Nuts including brazil, almond, walnut and cashew (enjoy as snacks)
- ✓ Nut butter - almond or cashew are particularly delicious
- ✓ Tahini Paste (use as a dip, adding lemon juice, salt, a dash of pepper or hot sauce for extra flavour). Pink Himalayan salt is the very best salt to use (from all health food shops)
- ✓ Avocados – great for breakfast, in a salad or smoothie
- ✓ Fish including fresh tuna, mackerel, salmon, herring, sardines, and trout
- ✓ If you can't or won't eat fish, look into a good quality fish oil supplement or Omega 3 Algae supplement
- ✓ Coconut oil or butter are the best oils to use for cooking
- ✓ Use olive oil, flaxseed oil and walnut oil over veg and salads

Did you know that healthy fats and oils help increase the chemical dopamine which is our motivation chemical?

Did you know that Tahini paste (made from pulped sesame seeds) has an excellent level of the mineral calcium? Good for those that don't eat dairy products.

Did you know that low-fat products often contain large amounts of sugar? A small, flavoured yoghurt can contain up to 8 teaspoons!

Did you know that burnt, trans and hydrogenated fats cause cell congestion so that nutrients cannot get into the cell as easily? Our bodies can't break down trans fats, so they act as toxins in the body! Hydrogen is added to the oil to give it a long shelf life, but our bodies can't break down these trans fats so they act as toxins in the body! We find trans fats in margarine as well as store bought biscuits, crackers, cakes, doughnuts, ready-made frozen pastry, frozen pizzas, microwave popcorn, and crisps. So check the ingredients for 'partially hydrogenated oils'. Some take-away restaurants also use hydrogenated oils for deep frying!

Water
Our bodies are about two-thirds water which is why it is recommended that we drink at least eight glasses of water every day. Water keeps our organs hydrated so they can function properly. It also helps to flush toxins and impurities out of your body. Dehydration affects the brain and can cause fuzzy thinking, poor concentration, low energy and feelings of hunger.

- ✓ Drink still water or for a treat fizzy water with an added slice of lemon or lime, ginger, mint, or even a piece of fruit!
- ✓ Drink fresh fruit juice diluted with water
- ✓ Calming, relaxing herbal teas include lemon balm, chamomile, peppermint and passionflower

✓ Energising herbal teas include apple, lemon and ginger, liquorice, green tea, and ginseng
✓ Eating hydrating foods such as fruit, vegetables and soups also helps

Sugar

Sugar is highly addictive and creates havoc with our health contributing to cancers, diabetes, heart disease, inflammatory and mood disorders. Natural sugar - found in whole grains, dairy, fruit and veg are what nature intended us to enjoy, but refined sugar is the problem and the fact that it is added to most processed foods. This last fact has led to a massive increase in obesity, particularly in the Western World. Personally, when I eat sugar, I find myself feeling not only anxious but sluggish and sleepy.

Consuming excess sugar:

✓ Reduces our immunity (it suppresses white blood cells)
✓ Reduces vitamins and minerals in our body
✓ Upsets hormones
✓ Upsets digestive processes
✓ Increases stress, anxiety and hyperactivity
✓ Increases cholesterol
✓ Increases fluid retention
✓ Increases ageing
✓ Increases weight gain
✓ Weakens eyesight
✓ Contributes to low blood sugar

Sugary foods and drinks can cause a roller coaster of high and low energy, high and low mood. When we eat refined, sugary foods it's like running a car on coke instead of petrol – not good quality fuel! Sugary foods, sugary drinks and refined carbs stimulate the fight/flight (stress response), so it is not just the boss, traffic jams or money worries which cause us to release stress hormones.

Reducing sugar can help us have a calmer mind, but avoid artificial sweeteners because research shows they cause intense cravings for sweets!

To help break the cycle and reduce sugar cravings:

- ✓ Eat protein at each meal
- ✓ Include some good fats (as noted above) in your daily diet
- ✓ Remove temptations from your kitchen
- ✓ Brush your teeth instead of reaching for something sweet – it works!
- ✓ Replace sugar with Xylitol - a natural sweetener which research shows is good for health, particularly for tooth cavities and blood sugar control
- ✓ Use a little honey initially to maintain some sweetness
- ✓ Snack on some veg sticks with a little tahini
- ✓ Snack on dates, a little dark chocolate, or a piece of Panda liquorice when cravings hit
- ✓ 1tsp L-Glutamine powder (an amino acid) can put a halt to sugar cravings. (I find that when I add glutamine to my whey protein smoothie, I feel much less drawn towards carbs of any kind!)
- ✓ The mineral chromium helps metabolise carbohydrates, fats and proteins and controls blood sugar. Anecdotal evidence suggests that chromium supplements can reduce cravings for refined carbohydrates and sugars and promote more stable sugar levels. Always take as part of a programme suggested by a Natural Health Practitioner.

Did you know eating sweet foods including sugary cereals in the first part of the day, tends to stimulate sweet cravings for the rest of the day, so the craving cycle continues?

Did you know that the average person in the USA and UK consumes roughly 20 - 30 teaspoons of added sugar per day in their tea, coffee, breakfast cereal, yoghurt, processed food, tinned food, ready meals, biscuits, sweets, alcohol and fizzy drinks?

Did you know that a can of coke has 7-8 teaspoons of sugar and that a packet of skittles has 8 teaspoons of sugar?

Did you know too much sugar and carby foods cause weight gain around the belly, known as belly fat?

Many of my clients who are on low protein diets have struggled with sugar cravings. When they up their protein content their cravings reduce.

When we feel more balanced and love ourselves more, sugar and junk food don't become so important to us (ongoing, ongoing!)

Think about what you really need in the moment:

- ✓ Is it a hug?
- ✓ Do you need to rest or sleep?
- ✓ Perhaps you need a rant to blow off some steam?
- ✓ Do you need to exercise or move your body?
- ✓ Do you need to express how you feel?

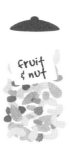

Chapter Seventeen

HEALTHY EATING TIPS

WHY do you want to make changes to your diet? To support a health condition?

To lose weight? To balance your emotions? To boost energy levels? To make sure your family are getting all the nutrients they need? Whatever the reason, setting a long-term goal is a fundamental component to keeping on track. Realise that food is nourishing your mind and body and then begin to make a few changes to build on over time.

Firstly, clean out your cupboards. Use up what you have, ready to re-stock with healthy staples, complimented by fresh ingredients.

Think swaps:

- ✓ Instead of sugary cereals for breakfast try:
    - eggs – boiled, poached, or scrambled and toast topped with avocado
    - natural yoghurt with chopped fresh or frozen fruit & seeds
    - creamy porridge
- ✓ Instead of bread try gluten free oatcakes or ryvita.
- ✓ Instead of regular pasta try rice noodles or quinoa.
- ✓ Instead of crisps have oatcakes with hummus.

- ✓ Instead of biscuits or cakes, try Naked Bars, Bounce Balls, raw nuts or fruit, and keep them on view.
- ✓ Carry healthy snacks to keep energy high and temptation at bay!
- ✓ Increase intake of water, green veg and whole grains.
- ✓ Reduce intake of sugar, fizzy drinks, and deep fried foods.

Learn to listen to your body's needs. Which foods make you feel good, and which make you feel tired or sluggish? What rhythm of eating works for you? Some people prefer to eat a substantial breakfast, a decent lunch and a small supper; others like to eat small meals and snack in between. Others have a schedule which requires their main meal at the end of the day.

Make a plan for you and your family that is workable. Keeping a daily food diary is extremely helpful for charting what you eat, and when, and note any symptoms that arise after eating specific foods. Like anything in life, changing your eating habits to create a healthier lifestyle has its ups and downs. Had a binge? Don't judge – it only causes stress – just accept, enjoy and get back on track! Are you opening a food cupboard out of boredom or for emotional reasons? Try substituting a slightly healthier option, or get out of the kitchen go for a walk, weed the garden, or call a friend!

- ✓ Shop for healthy options that you can mix and match to create a meal that doesn't involve much cooking: boiled eggs, smoked salmon, feta cheese, olives, oatcakes, cherry tomatoes, avocados, tinned fish or beans.
- ✓ Cook soups, stews and casseroles in bulk and freeze to save cooking daily.
- ✓ Eat fruit and veg in a rainbow of colours to take advantage of the full range of vitamins, minerals and antioxidants.

- ✓ Use seasonal, locally grown produce where possible.
- ✓ Gradually introduce new foods.
- ✓ Treat yourself to a cookbook and check out recipes online.
- ✓ Make a list of ideas for appealing meals you'd like to prepare.
- ✓ Involve the family in cooking and making smoothies together.
- ✓ Look for healthier versions of ready meals in supermarkets and shops.
- ✓ Look for cafés that make healthy homemade soups and salads.
- ✓ Enjoy your treats. Don't feel guilty – but do remember that they are treats!

Spice Up Your Life - Well Your Food Anyway!

Herbs and spices have health benefits as well as adding flavour! Enjoy them in soups, curries, stews, dahl, smoothies, on fish and roast veg.

- ✓ Nutmeg & ginger (good for digestive health)
- ✓ Sage, coriander & cinnamon (aid blood sugar control and fat burning)
- ✓ Mint, basil & turmeric (help reduce inflammation and pain)
- ✓ Rosemary (good for memory)
- ✓ Cayenne Pepper (helps improve circulation)
- ✓ Parsley (like a multivitamin)

Look after your body well. It is your vehicle for life.

> *"A man too busy to take care of his health*
> *is like a mechanic too busy to take care of his tools."*
> *Spanish Proverb*

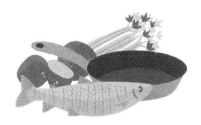

Chapter Eighteen

A HEALTHY MIND AND BODY

A HEALTHY internal environment helps us cope with invading bugs, viruses and illness. Toxins, processed, junk and sugary food, as well as a stressful lifestyle, affect our health and wellbeing negatively, creating the potential to develop diseases. It's also important to realise that all bodily systems are interrelated and work together to promote our health. If one organ or system is knocked off, it can affect others. For instance, a toxic or sluggish liver can affect female hormones, digestion and your skin.

We can look after our health by feeding ourselves nutritious food, by drinking filtered water and enjoying fresh air and exercise. Other essential components include supportive relationships, love, laughter and having a passion or two in life!

While my ME/CFS was triggered by vaccinations and glandular fever, I now know that my internal environment and immune system weren't in the best of health due to years of stress, antibiotics, wrong food and a lack of direction. There is no judgement - only understanding now.

Blood Sugar

Balancing blood sugar is a vital factor in keeping healthy. Blood sugar refers to the levels of glucose in the blood, the primary source of energy for your cells. After eating unrefined food, blood sugar rises gradually and gently reduces until we eat again. With balanced blood sugar levels our energy, concentration, moods and emotions are good. Too much stress, caffeine, sugary foods and drinks, refined carbohydrates, low protein intake, and junk food, cause blood sugar highs and lows. These fluctuations lead to unstable energy, uneven emotions, anger, anxiety and a reduced ability to cope with stress. It also sets up a cycle of cravings.

Overeating carbohydrates, skipping meals and snacking on chocolates and biscuits cause highs and lows and is one of the first things I discuss with clients.

Blood sugar levels are lower in the morning, and if you miss breakfast, they will be even lower. When blood sugar drops too low (hypoglycaemia) you can experience shaking, anxiety, poor concentration, cravings, irritability and headaches to name a few. This can also cause migraines IBS or PMS to flare up.

Insulin is the key that unlocks cells to allow glucose to enter. When we eat too many carby or sugary foods and drinks it overproduces. If the mechanism is severely overworked, the cells actively resist the insulin so that the glucose stays in the blood. Glucose in the blood turns to fat and can eventually leads to diabetes. Too much glucose (sugar) in the blood is highly toxic both to the body and brain.

Tips for Balancing Blood Sugar Levels
- ✓ Eat regular meals
- ✓ Eat a protein rich breakfast
- ✓ Eat protein with each meal: lean meat, fish, cheese, natural yoghurt, beans, lentils, nuts, seeds. (Protein helps us feel full and slows sugar release)

✓ Choose healthy fats found in oily fish, nuts, seeds, coconut oil, and avocados

✓ Choose complex carbohydrates: whole grain pasta and bread, oats, brown or wild rice, quinoa, sweet potatoes. Reduce grains overall

✓ Greatly reduce sugary foods and white carbs

✓ Reduce drinks which spike blood sugar and result in a crash an hour or so later: alcohol, caffeine, sugary drinks and energy drinks

✓ Record your caffeine, chocolate and alcohol intake!

✓ We all have different tolerance levels. Caffeine can temporarily lift our mood, concentration and energy, but for many it's followed by an energy crash, cravings and irritability. Caffeine is found in tea, coffee, chocolate, energy drinks, 'flu remedies and painkillers. Look in health food shops for caffeine alternatives e.g. Barleycup.

Did you know that:

✓ Caffeine and sugar can disrupt sleep patterns?

✓ Feeling stressed can cause us to eat more sugar – which makes us feel even more panicked and wired?

✓ White refined carbs and sugar can act like a drug?

✓ We only need one tsp of sugar/glucose in the blood at any one time to balance hormones and energy?

✓ Some people who eat a high carb lunch feel sleepy shortly afterwards?

If you wake between 2-3 am, it can indicate that your blood sugar has dropped too low. The adrenalin produced can cause restless legs, anxiety or hunger. Have a snack before bed to prevent this happening: ½ an apple and some nuts, or an oatcake spread with nut butter. During the night you could eat an oatcake and a few nuts to help you get back to sleep.

	Upsetting Blood Sugar	Balancing Blood Sugar
Breakfast	Coffee and croissant Sugary cereal, toast and jam	Scrambled egg with veg and avocado Sugar-free muesli Porridge with berries, natural yoghurt, nuts and seeds
Lunch	White bread sandwich, chocolate bar and fizzy drink	Chicken/Fish/Egg/Bean salad with soup Whole grain sandwich Oatcakes with cold meat and salad
Dinner	White pasta with tomato sauce and garlic bread	Turkey and butter bean curry Stew with sweet potatoes Salmon with veg and wild rice Omelette with veg/salad
Snacks	Crisps, chocolate, biscuits, fizzy juice, coffee, cereal bars	Fruit and nuts/seeds Oatcakes with topping Boiled egg

Stress

Our bodies have developed our 'fight or flight' response over millions of years. In hunter-gatherer days, people sometimes had to face a sabre-tooth tiger! Yet, they lived in a close-knit tribal environment with social support and spiritual guidance from elders. A situation very different from today's fast-paced life which offers less and less community support with our bodies reacting in the same way to money worries, unresolved emotional issues, a bullying boss, ongoing inflammation, or illness, to a life threatening situation like a sabre tooth tiger! Traffic jams, lack of sleep, shift work, poor diet (such as sugary, junk and processed foods), toxins, busy lifestyles, juggling work and childcare, technology, fear, over-thinking, injury, and a chemically charged environment all cause us low-level stress with that age-old fight or flight reaction.

We are running on overdrive, out of balance with our bodies and nature, putting immense pressure on our adrenal glands. These tiny glands, which sit just above our kidneys, help control our blood sugar, blood pressure, response to stress, inflammation, immune response and balance female hormones necessary for fertility. So when our adrenal glands have been under too much pressure, we can suffer burn-out! Many people today can feel stuck in fight or flight mode.

Our own reactions to stress vary due to genetics, upbringing, experiences and personal characteristics. Symptoms of stress and adrenal fatigue can range from allergies, anxiety, back pain, catching colds and 'flu, cravings, poor concentration, low mood, difficulty losing weight, digestive problems, fatigue, headaches, hormonal imbalances, inflammation, insomnia, joint pain, low self-esteem, muscle tension, feeling run down, feeling wired all the time. IBS and other symptoms can also flare up or worsen when we are stressed. And remember that when we are under stress, we are inclined to eat sugary foods to gear up for fighting or fleeing that sabre-tooth tiger! In the same way, we turn to comfort food when our stressed selves feel unhappy, lonely, tired or low. We rarely crave a carrot when we are stressed!

A healthy diet, balancing your blood sugar, relaxation techniques and regular exercise is highly beneficial for beating stress. When we strengthen, support, calm and cleanse the body with good food, supplements, relaxation, mindfulness and exercise we can become more resilient to day to day life and cope better.

Did you know that magnesium found in dark chocolate, green leafy veg, nuts, seeds, fish, avocados and whole grains is known as nature's tranquilliser?

Other foods and nutrients to support stress and the adrenals - from the anti-stress 'calm' larder include:

- ✓ Vitamin C rich foods found in fresh fruit and veg – try kiwi, tomatoes, strawberries, peppers, cauliflower, raspberries, cherries, oranges
- ✓ Whole grains such as oats, brown wheat germ, brown rice, quinoa – have many stress busting B vitamins as does lean meat, eggs and dairy products
- ✓ Green leafy veg such as spinach kale, celery and broccoli, watercress – rich in calcium and magnesium which have a calming effect on the body
- ✓ Natural yoghurt
- ✓ Whey protein
- ✓ Oily fish, prawns, shellfish
- ✓ Avocados
- ✓ Kidney beans, aduki beans, celery
- ✓ Sweet potatoes
- ✓ Nuts, such as almonds and brazils
- ✓ Sunflower seeds
- ✓ Bananas
- ✓ Blueberries

- ✓ Small amounts of dark chocolate
- ✓ Nettle tea, rosehip tea
- ✓ Calming teas such as chamomile, lavender, passionflower, lemon balm, valerian
- ✓ Green tea – has a component L-Theanine which is calming
- ✓ GABA is a calming chemical in the brain, made from glutamine found in meat, milk, yoghurt, spinach, tomatoes and cabbage

Chapter Eleven has suggestions on how to deal with stress. Try to be honest with yourself about what you can achieve in a day. Prioritise. Don't take on too much. Share feelings and get support by seeing your GP, a counsellor, or therapist.

Female Hormones

This finely tuned and delicate system can be affected by stress, illness, medication, poor diet, excess caffeine, alcohol and toxins in the environment, pregnancy, and childbirth. I have suffered from PMS, fertility issues, and experienced hormonal imbalances including after the birth of Sophia. My hormones crashed when Sophia was about 10 months old and I took bio-identical progesterone cream for some time which helped a great deal. New research is coming out on post natal burn-out which can occur months or even years later! Hormonal imbalances can result in issues such as mood swings, anxiety, heavy bleeding, infertility, period problems and even Polycystic Ovarian Syndrome.

A low processed, high wholefood diet including fruit, veg, lean proteins, pulses, seeds, nuts and good fats helps balance and support these hormones. Some especially beneficial foods are ground flaxseeds, brown rice, oats, walnuts, chickpeas, lentils, coconut oil, broccoli, cabbage and kale. Balancing blood sugar as above is vital to help stabilise your hormones. Trans fats, deep fried fats, excess caffeine, sugar and alcohol all upset our hormonal balance.

I have read that when serotonin naturally lowers before menstruation, it can cause water retention. So balancing blood sugar by eating well can help water retention by regulating serotonin levels. WOW!

Did you know when we crave chocolate before our period, it could indicate a magnesium deficiency – a mineral that supports our hormones and blood sugar among other tasks, and that is found in chocolate?

Did you know that oestrogen stimulates serotonin our feel good chemical and helps block excess of the stress hormone cortisol? Because oestrogen levels drop before a period (and during menopause), it's one reason why we feel less able to cope. Our central nervous system is highly sensitive to hormonal fluctuations, which affects mood and anxiety levels, another reason why we can feel anxious or low for no apparent reason?

Did you know that ground flaxseeds, as well as being a rich source of Omega 3 oils, are high in fibre which helps clear old toxic hormones which are no longer needed?

As I am just entering the peri-menopausal phase of my life I am aware that many fear this natural stage. Yet, if you put yourself first, look at your stress, and try meditating, as well as eating well to create a well-adjusted lifestyle, you can help support a happier transition to mark a new positive beginning in many ways. The hormone progesterone is particularly helpful during the menopause to maintain blood sugar levels and calm the mind and body among other functions. Acupuncture and the use of herbs are also good ways of supporting hormonal health. This can all apply to male hormones too. I'd also like to mention the benefit of using natural cleaning products and personal self-care products, as the chemicals in regular products can also disrupt this delicate hormonal system.

Immunity

There is still much to learn about our amazing immune systems, but their role is to defend and protect our bodies against infections, viruses, cancer cells, inflammation, fungi and parasites. Your immune system is not located in any one part of your body but throughout it – for example, the mucous membranes in your mouth and nose, your liver, your gut, your blood (e.g. white cells, macrophages) and lymph. It is the health of our 'internal terrain' which helps keep us well. Weak immunity can also contribute to fatigue and allergies.

We all get sick from time to time, and our immune systems help us get well again. However, there are many factors which deplete the function of our immune systems such as stress, chronic infections, poor diet, antibiotics, excess sugar, poor digestion, toxic overload and low levels of nutrients.

Foods which support our immune system include:

- ✓ Lean meat, fish, eggs, beans, lentils, oats, brown rice, quinoa
- ✓ Fruit and veg such as sweet potatoes, kiwi, berries, carrots, peppers
- ✓ Avocados, coconut oil and milk, asparagus, broccoli, onions, leeks, shitake mushrooms
- ✓ Dark chocolate, cinnamon, ginger, garlic, cayenne pepper, turmeric
- ✓ Drink plenty of fluids
- ✓ Reduce sugary food, processed and junk food. Refined sugar can feed viruses, parasites and fungi in the body and deplete essential nutrients

Get out your slow cooker and make delicious, nourishing stews and casseroles and homemade soups to help keep your body warm.

Other factors which enhance immune health are:

- ✓ Rest and sleep.
- ✓ Epsom Salt baths are a lovely way to gently detox and relax due to their magnesium content. Also helpful if you feel a cold coming. Buy from health food shops or online.
- ✓ Meditation, yoga, tai chi, laughter, close relationships, massage, gratitude, fresh air.
- ✓ Good quality supplements can help boost and support immunity: Vitamin D, Vitamin C, Zinc, Magnesium, Elderberry, Echinacea, Probiotics, Beta Glucans, Omega 3 oils – but always check with your GP or Nutritional Therapist if on medication.

Health Tip

If you do succumb to bugs, wrap up warm, drink plenty of fluids, gargle with salt water or tea tree oil, and have a hot toddy. Make a healing soup from red onions, garlic, carrots, sweet potato, fresh ginger, turmeric, stock and coconut milk. Puree and serve with love! Relax and let your body heal. Remember one or two colds a year can actually be a good thing. It is your body`s way of clearing out wastes and toxins which build up inside. Runny nose, eyes and a temperature are natural ways the body detoxes and heals.

Digestion

Your digestive system runs from your mouth to your anus. If your gut isn't happy, you won't feel right or energised. Your digestive system plays a vital role in keeping you healthy. It helps protect against invaders. It prepares, digests and absorbs nutrients from your food. It also eliminates waste products. Your digestive system can be upset or weakened by stress and worry;

antibiotics and medicines; infection; illness; lack of exercise; food poisoning; and too much processed, fatty or acidic food. There are many supplements specifically aimed to support digestion. These include aloe vera, slippery elm, probiotics, digestive enzymes, L-Glutamine and zinc.

Tips to Improve Digestive Health

- ✓ Drink a mug of warm water with lemon juice first thing in the morning. It helps cleanse left over waste from your gut.
- ✓ All digestion starts in the mouth so really chew your food well – your stomach doesn`t have teeth!
- ✓ Try taking a tablespoon of apple cider vinegar in warm water before food to aid your digestion.
- ✓ Take time out to eat, away from the computer, the car or in the street!
- ✓ Try to relax a bit before eating because when we are stressed or in a hurry, the body diverts energy away from digestion, which is why we bloat or get indigestion.
- ✓ Sitting down to eat is also important, but avoid slumping!
- ✓ Try mindful eating - turn off distractions, sit down, slow down, savour, enjoy, be present!
- ✓ Eat wholefoods from nature - the body can't digest processed foods easily.
- ✓ Fruit, veg and fibre are good for your digestion: carrots, sweet potatoes, squash, avocado, mango and stewed apples.
- ✓ Onions, garlic, leeks, artichokes, oats, flaxseeds and barley feed the friendly bacteria in our gut.
- ✓ Fish and white meat are easier to digest than red meat.
- ✓ Don't overeat - the body uses vast amounts of energy to digest food which is why we often feel sleepy or tired after a big meal.

- ✓ Eat smaller, simpler meals - fish with sweet potato and green beans, or chicken with asparagus and broccoli.
- ✓ One pot meals help break down the meats which also helps.
- ✓ Once you have eaten your meal, it's a good idea to sit for at least 5 minutes before rushing off to your next task!
- ✓ Why not have a cup of fennel, peppermint, dandelion and nettle herbal tea to aid digestion first.
- ✓ Eat regular meals.
- ✓ Try making bone broth which supports gut health and healing.
- ✓ Take probiotics and eat some fermented foods such as sauerkraut.
- ✓ Supporting your liver also helps (see next section).

Did you know that 60-70% of your immune system is located in your gut which is why a strong, healthy gut can enhance overall health?

Did you know that according to latest medical research you have two brains - one in your head and the other in your gut!? The two brains talk to each through the nervous system. So what one brain feels so will the other. Think butterflies in your stomach when you feel anxious or stressed. Think of the headache that you get when you haven't drunk enough water or eaten all day. Or irritation or low mood if you eat too much junk food or foods to which you are intolerant.

My daughter, Sophia often goes on about good and bad guys in cartoons! One of the good guys for our health are the friendly bacteria found in our guts. Also, supplementing with probiotics aids digestion and absorption of nutrients, helps prevent diarrhoea and symptoms of food poisoning and IBS. These beneficial bacteria also support immunity, allergies, food intolerances, weight, urinary health, hormonal health, cholesterol, mood and emotional health. Amazing really! (Probiotics literally means 'promotion of life'.)

Friendly health promoting bacteria can become depleted through stress, surgery, old age, a diet of processed food, little fibre, too much alcohol and sugary food, antibiotics and other medications, pollution and chemicals. So taking a digestive enzyme or probiotic supplement before eating can make a difference to your well-being.

Liver Health

The liver is an amazing organ that performs many essential functions. It absorbs and stores nutrients; helps control blood sugar levels, produces bile to help digest fats; clears out wastes and toxins, and controls cholesterol levels.

Our liver is put under stress when we take in too much sugar, alcohol, caffeine, medication, processed food, and are surrounded by an environment overloaded with chemicals and toxins. Symptoms may include skin problems, low energy, depressed mood, aches and pains, difficulty losing weight, headaches, foggy head, allergies and IBS.

My liver has suffered twice. Once from all the antibiotics I took when I had ME, and secondly when I had Glandular Fever which affects the liver's ability to digest and process fats. I'm so glad I took up nutrition!

A wholefood diet helps support your liver:

- ✓ Drink water, nettle and dandelion teas.
- ✓ Eat asparagus, avocados, beetroot, berries, broccoli, brown rice, carrots, cucumber, eggs, leafy greens, oily fish, radishes, and walnuts.
- ✓ Reduce sugary foods and drinks, wheat, deep fried foods, alcohol, fatty meats and cheeses.
- ✓ Take B vitamins, milk thistle and artichoke.

✓ Lecithin granules sprinkled on cereal, in yoghurt or smoothies help to cleanse the liver and break down fats.

Weight Balancing

There are many factors which explain the startling rise in obesity over the last few decades from toxic environments to pollution, pesticides, and plastics, to hormone disrupting chemicals and food additives. We have 24-hour supermarkets offering highly processed and sugar-laden foods, takeaways offering food laden with bad fats, and restaurants offering huge portion sizes. Longer, stressful working hours are also curtailing time to cook healthy meals and spend time out in nature to breathe clean oxygen and recharge.

It is important to think lifestyle change rather than embarking on a 'diet'. I never recommend calorie counting, low-fat diets, self-denial, or obsessive dieting. They tend to lead to a drop in energy and mood, which in turn leads to comfort eating, guilt, and self-loathing! While the right foods in reasonable amounts are vital, so too is finding physical, mental and emotional balance. When my clients find equilibrium in their lives, they usually find that their weight stabilises!

Did you know that calorie counting doesn't take into account the quality of the food? A steak and a chocolate bar can have similar calorific values, but guess which one would result in stored fat – the chocolate bar!

Did you know that it's not only food and exercise that affects our weight and our ability to shift the pounds? Our bodies are less able to metabolise food and burn fat when we are ill or taking medication; have suppressed hormonal, vitamin, mineral and gut bacteria levels; or are under that little word, stress!

Did you know that heightened stress levels secrete the hormone cortisol which not only increases appetite but can also result in stored abdominal fat?

Did you know that stress also lowers serotonin levels – the feel good hormone which helps curb carb cravings?

Tips to Help Balance Weight

- ✓ Support your digestion and your liver (as above).
- ✓ Take probiotics, B vitamins, chromium, magnesium & Vitamin D.
- ✓ Include chai seeds, flax seeds, spirulina and walnuts in your daily diet.
- ✓ Eat real food rather than processed food.
- ✓ Eat a protein rich breakfast.
- ✓ Chew your food really well.
- ✓ Stop eating before you feel full.
- ✓ Make fresh soups. They are chock full of nutrients and fill you up.
- ✓ Remember to have healthy snacks in between meals: protein balls, nuts, avocado, tahini or hummus on oat cakes and ryvita.
- ✓ Have protein, good fats, and non-starchy veg with each meal - the foods which have less effect on insulin levels. (Remember the more insulin you produce, the more the body is primed to store food as fat!)
- ✓ Swap sugary foods for berries, dates or dark chocolate (75%).
- ✓ Swap refined carbohydrates for brown rice, quinoa and millet.
- ✓ Replace supermarket household and self-care goods with natural products.
- ✓ Increase relaxation - try mindfulness or meditation.
- ✓ Make time for exercise – something you enjoy be it walking, yoga, martial arts or dancing, Pilates or pumping iron!
- ✓ Love and accept yourself how you are now

We don't need to be perfect all the time! Eating well is beneficial to our wellbeing, but be sure to savour and enjoy treats – be they a glass of wine, cake, or a bar of chocolate. Just don't go mad with them! Health is about more than a number on the scales, perfect abs, a body like those on magazine covers, or eating perfectly 100% of the time. When we allow ourselves a little leeway without guilt, we naturally want to eat healthy foods the rest of the time.

Over time we can start listening to our intuition and body signals regarding what foods feel right for us. You may get a 'craving' for vegetables if you have been eating too many processed foods!

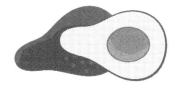

Chapter Nineteen

FOOD, MOOD AND THE BRAIN

I AM particularly interested in the way food influences our mood. Did you know that while a healthy diet supports brain health and protects the brain cells, specific foods can help boost concentration, memory and learning?

The brain is a sensitive organ and the effects of food on mood are an important part of the mental health jigsaw alongside lifestyle, stress, modern life, social and environmental factors, support networks, coping strategies and personality. Once again a natural, wholefood diet boosts mood and brain function. Slow release carbs, healthy fats, plenty of fluids and a rainbow of fruit and veg. Sardines, egg yolk, organ meats, Brazil nuts and walnuts, as well as lecithin granules, also help enhance mood, brain communication and memory.

Avoid additives and preservatives such as E-numbers and MSG. Also stay away from artificial sweeteners such as sucralose, saccharin, (aspartame), acesulfame K, and neotame which are often present in ready meals, low-fat products, soft drinks, and sugar-free products. So check the ingredients of any processed foods because the presence of these chemicals numb our thinking and can contribute to low mood, anxiety, irritability, and increase sugar cravings.

Excess caffeine can also overstimulate the central nervous system, increase palpitations, anxiety, insomnia, irritation and upset blood sugar levels. Did you know that one cup of coffee can increase stress hormone cortisol up to 30% for as long as an hour! No wonder some people feel wired, anxious or stressed after drinking coffee!

Neurotransmitters are the brain chemicals that communicate information throughout the brain and body. They instruct the heart to beat and the stomach to digest. These chemicals influence sleep, concentration, mood and the way we think and feel but are affected by what we eat and drink. New research shows that inflammation in the body due to stress, toxins, processed food and junk food affects your brain and your mood as well as your joints. So cleaning up your diet reduces inflammation in the body and the brain.

Serotonin

This brain chemical (which is also found in the gut and other areas in the body) enables us to feel calmer, happier, increases self-esteem, boosts mood, aids sleep and reduces cravings. Low levels can lead to anxiety, OCD, depression, low self-esteem, lower pain threshold, impulsive behaviour and cravings for sugar and alcohol. Modern living, multi-tasking, stress as well as being indoors can deplete serotonin levels. Another factor which can reduce serotonin is too much bacteria and yeast in our gut which is caused by overeating sugars and carbohydrates.

Foods which can help boost serotonin levels include fish, turkey, chicken, cottage cheese, bananas, eggs, nuts, seeds, whey protein, veg and slow release carbs such as oats and brown rice. Exercise, natural light and lowering stress levels help boost serotonin.

Did you know essential (good) fats help boost levels of serotonin? Many people today have diets low in these essential fats which can be a contributing factor to low mood. Try cooking with coconut oil, and adding avocados and oily fish such as mackerel and salmon to your diet and be sure to dress your salads with extra virgin olive oil – another good fat.

Did you know that meditation can increase serotonin levels? Another reason to take time out and breathe!

Dopamine and Noradrenalin

These are neurotransmitters that help us stay awake and motivated. To boost their levels, eat meat, chicken, salmon, beans, cheese, and nuts, bananas, avocados and seeds as well as healthy fats. And remember, too many carbs at lunchtime can make us sleepy!

Endorphins

Beta-Endorphins are chemicals produced in our body and brain that help enhance mood and create feelings of relaxation and well-being. Symptoms of low beta-endorphins include low pain tolerance, low self-esteem, feeling tearful, depressed, emotional and overwhelmed as well as craving sugar and carbs. Sugar and alcohol can temporarily increase beta-endorphins, but there is a resulting vicious cycle of high and low spikes upsetting mood and wellbeing.

Activities that increase beta-endorphins naturally include:

- ✓ Meditation
- ✓ Exercise
- ✓ Music
- ✓ Fun
- ✓ Watching a feel-good movie
- ✓ Dancing
- ✓ Being out in the fresh air

- ✓ Browsing in a store you love
- ✓ Orgasm!
- ✓ Inspirational talks
- ✓ Yoga
- ✓ Good Food
- ✓ Prayer
- ✓ Stroking a pet
- ✓ Reading a book or magazine
- ✓ Massage
- ✓ People/places/animals you love

Try to do something you enjoy each day to help raise your mood and combat stress.

Once again, balancing your blood sugar levels contributes to maintaining a balance of feel good brain chemicals, and you can do this by:

- ✓ Eating regular meals
- ✓ Eating a protein rich breakfast
- ✓ Eating protein with each meal such as lean meat, fish, cheese, natural yoghurt, beans, lentils, nuts, seeds. Protein helps us feel full and slows sugar release
- ✓ Choose good fats found in oily fish, nuts, seeds, coconut oil, and avocados
- ✓ Choosing complex carbohydrates: whole grain pasta and bread, oats, brown or wild rice, quinoa, sweet potatoes
- ✓ Reducing drinks which spike blood sugar and result in a crash an hour or so later: alcohol, caffeine, sugary drinks, and energy drinks

Did you know that chocolate contains sugar, stimulants and endorphin enhancing chemicals which is why it is so pleasurable and addictive? It affects brain chemicals that control mood, behaviour and mental function. Eating dark chocolate with a cacao content of 75% or higher is much better for you and it contains much less sugar and other additives. Also 'raw' chocolate which you can either buy ready made at health food shops or make yourself. You can purchase a kit for making raw chocolate online from www.elementsforlife.co.uk.

Omega 3 Fatty Acids

These are essential for maintaining a good mood and good behaviour as well as assisting learning and brain health. A study in the 2016 British Journal of Nutrition suggests how Omega 3 oils are important for mood and brain function. The study details how Omega 3 oils are important for brain structure and support the transmission of messages between cells in the brain and nervous system. Without sufficient Omega 3 fats, cell communication can become crackly and interrupted. So it is recommended to eat 2-3 portions of oily fish per week and / or take fish oil supplements. Vegetarians can take chia seeds, hemp seeds, pumpkin seeds, walnuts and Omega 3 rich eggs and algae supplements which are rich in Omega 3 fatty acids.

Did you know Omega 3 helps build and maintain the myelin sheath, (which helps keep nerve fibres insulated) so messages can flow better between cells?

Did you know that for many people reducing sugar and gluten (found in wheat products) can increase peace in the brain? In some people, too much gluten can negatively affect serotonin levels.

A Little Bit On Anxiety

Anxiety and panic attacks can be aggravated by food and drink which trigger stress hormones or upset blood sugar levels. Often, these foods are the ones we crave in times of stress: alcohol, sugary foods, cakes, chocolate bars, processed and refined carbs, and caffeine. Typical, I know!

One of my clients who switched to using decaff tea and coffee continued to experience palpitations until she cut them out completely – so be aware that decaff coffee, tea and green tea still contain small amounts of caffeine. Tune into your body to see how your food and drink intake is affecting you. We are all different!

Did you know that maintaining good gut bacteria supports mood and anxiety as well as enhancing digestion and immunity? Taking probiotics can calm the gut which in turn can help calm the brain. So taking a good probiotic can be invaluable for maintaining overall brain and body health,

Coping with Food Sensitivity and Allergies

People are reacting to milk, wheat, soya, corn, sugar, eggs, and yeast these days. Symptoms might include diarrhoea, stomach cramps, sinus congestion, anxiety, mood issues and poor concentration which usually manifest from an hour after eating or drinking, to as long as three days later. Allergic symptoms are entirely different. They often manifest as a rash, asthma, eczema, or a swelling of the mouth or throat. Some people find that they experience rashes, headaches and irritability after drinking red wine, eating smoked fish or meat, sausages, cheese and chocolate – all of which contain a substance known as 'amines'. If that is the case, it is best to avoid all of them. I highly recommend varying the foods you eat so that you are not eating the same thing day in day out. Also, try keeping a food diary to make a note of how you feel after eating certain foods. If you eat cereal or toast for breakfast, a sandwich for lunch and then pasta for dinner - that's wheat three times a day!

If wheat or gluten is an issue in your life, leave out bread and try substituting rice cakes or oatcakes (which have much less gluten). You can also find gluten free bread and tortillas. A note of warning here - gluten free cakes and biscuits tend to have lots of added sugar, so do check the ingredients! You can also purchase gluten free muesli and pasta. However, spiralising courgettes to top with your favourite pasta sauce has gained a huge following and is well worth trying. As is cauliflower rice!

If you want to accompany your meal with a carbohydrate, try rice noodles, quinoa or millet. Jacket potatoes and sweet potatoes are also good alternatives - try some baked sweet potato slices or chunks, with coconut oil and herbs or salt. Delicious! If dairy is a problem, instead of cow's milk try sheep's or goat's milk, oat or rice milk, sugar-free almond or coconut milk. Rather than using bought salad dressings which have additives, make your own from olive oil and balsamic vinegar or apple cider vinegar, or lemon juice. You can add herbs, spices, garlic and mustard. It's great to experiment to find the one you love. Instead of purchasing fizzy or energy drinks which are full of additives and sugar, sugar substitutes and caffeine, try fizzy water with a slice of lemon, or a little elderflower cordial. Or buy coconut water which is packed full of goodness.

Food Cravings
You can have a physical craving when your stomach feels empty or if you are suffering from a mineral deficiency. When you have strong emotions be they angry, happy or sad, the body often looks to food for comfort. Or you might have just got into a habit - always reaching for a specific unhealthy snack at a particular time of day. You might be eating a diet lacking in fresh food and laden with chemicals, and the body is signalling the brain that it needs a pick-me-up. Cravings can also mean that the body has got its signals mixed. You might be feeling exhausted, stressed, dehydrated, anxious or have low blood sugar.

Happy Snacks

✓ Oatcakes or Veg Sticks with
  hummus, nut butter or avocado
✓ Apple Slices with Tahini
  or Sugar-Free Peanut Butter
✓ Coconut Chunks / Nuts / Fruit
✓ Dark chocolate
✓ Energy Balls
✓ Flapjacks w/dried fruit and oats
✓ Sparkling Water
✓ Herbal Teas
✓ Coconut Water

Sad Snacks

✓ Chips
✓ Crisps
✓ Tortilla Chips
✓ Pork Scratchings
✓ Donuts
✓ Milk Chocolate
✓ Sweets
✓ Sugary Cereal Bars
✓ Fizzy Drinks
✓ Caffeinated Tea
✓ Caffeinated Coffee

Cravings tend toward chocolate, carbs, crisps, chips, salty food, pizza or alcohol. Any one of those foods will give you a short burst of energy and lift of mood, followed by a crash which initiates the craving cycle all over again.

Did you know we sometimes crave the foods which we are sensitive to - such as the milk in milk chocolate?

When we feel stressed, tired, bored or low, this affects our ability to make better food choices. So food and mood is a 2-way process.

Processed and chemical laden food can temporarily increase our feel-good hormones. For some people, even the casein found in milk products provides a kind of high not unlike opiates!

Some Tips to Help with Cravings
  ✓ Remove temptations from the house or office!

✓ Have healthy foods in the house.

✓ Introduce more good quality protein and fats into your diet

✓ Take L-Glutamine daily. It helps reduce cravings for sugar and alcohol.

✓ When you are 'craving' something, wait 10 minutes to see if it passes.

✓ Try drinking a glass of water as cravings are often due to dehydration.

✓ Start an activity or take a walk.

✓ If you are in the midst of a strong emotion breathe in for 7 and out for 11 for five minutes – it calms you right down, and you will feel much better.

✓ Remove yourself from an area where food is present but if you really need a snack, eat a healthy one! Or ones that are much lower in sugar.

✓ Hypnotherapy can help.

Did you know it takes about 21 days to break a habit? It can also take time for taste buds to adjust and thoroughly enjoy new flavours.

Supplements which can help support mood and brain health include:

✓ 5-HTP, St Johns Wort, Taurine, Tyrosine, L-Theanine, L-Glutamine

✓ Rhodiola, Ashwagandha, Lemon Balm, Valerian, Chamomile

✓ Fish oils, Magnesium, B Vitamins, Zinc, Chromium, Iron, Antioxidants

✓ Phosphatidyle serine and Phospahatidyle choline

Booking a session with a Nutritional Therapist is best to create a programme especially tailored for you. Always check with your GP if you have a health condition or are taking medication.

Meals to Support Brain Health and Mood

Breakfast

Porridge with Berries, Cinnamon, Natural Yoghurt, Walnuts and Almonds: Oats are slow release carbs/Berries are full of nutrients, and antioxidants/Cinnamon helps support blood sugar/Natural yoghurt has protein/Nuts have healthy fats, vitamins and minerals including magnesium and zinc.

Lunch

Mug of Homemade Soup plus Boiled Egg Salad with Avocado, Salad Leaves, Olives, Tomato and Cucumber:

Eggs are rich in protein, and the nutrient choline important for mood and memory/Avocado and Olives contain beneficial fats to help lubricate the brain/Salad and Soup boost levels of magnesium, calcium, B vitamins, beta-carotene and Vitamin C.

Dinner

Baked Salmon Steak with Sweet Potato Wedges and Steamed Broccoli: Salmon is full of Omega 3 fats vital for brain health, and mood/ Sweet Potatoes are rich in fibre, slow release carbs, as well as magnesium, folic acid and Vitamin E/Broccoli, contains protective antioxidants plus calcium, magnesium and B vitamins.

Tips for a More Balanced Lifestyle
- ✓ Natural therapies such as Acupuncture, Reiki, Reflexology, Massage, Herbs, Flower Essences, Essential Oils.

- ✓ Nature, Fresh Air.
- ✓ Sleeping, Resting, Slowing Down.
- ✓ Take the pressure off yourself by Saying No!
- ✓ Yoga, Pilates, Tai Chi.
- ✓ Breathing, Meditation, Mindfulness, Visualisation.
- ✓ Epsom Salt Baths.
- ✓ Purpose, Passion, Meaning, Fun, Music, Creativity, Volunteer Work.
- ✓ Take a Digital Detox: an hour, or even a day away from gadgets and phones. Take a break from harmful EMF's which emit from digital equipment.
- ✓ Purchase Orgonite to protect you from EMF's.
- ✓ Remove mobile phones and computers from the bedroom while you sleep.

Listen to your intuition, to what your body needs, to what activities you'd like to try. Try not take everything so seriously and have a bit more fun. I know I can be way too serious sometimes about myself and life! Be silly! Dance, laugh, watch a funny video clip. It truly benefits your health to lighten up! Find something you enjoy doing that helps you relax and incorporate it into your daily life. Play an instrument, take up painting, knitting or cross-stitch, join a skittles or tennis club! My client David enjoys cooking and finds that helps him to relax.

Focused activities take our attention away from problems and responsibilities, relaxing the mind and soothing the amygdala that mobilises our fight or flight mode.

In our fast paced lives, we forget to make time for ourselves. Perhaps we feel guilty if we aren't working, or helping others, but it is vital for our health and wellbeing to take the time to nurture ourselves.

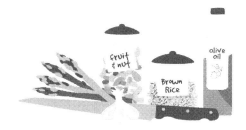

Chapter Twenty

SUPERFOODS AND STOCKING THE LARDER

THERE are many foodstuffs touted as the latest superfood – from chai seeds and goji berries to acai berries. Here are ten nutritious day-to-day superfoods I eat regularly – what are yours?

Almonds and Walnuts – Nutty and Good for You!
Help support cardiovascular health, blood sugar, bone health, metabolism, brain and mood. Rich in antioxidants, magnesium, calcium, potassium, zinc, Omega 3 and 6 essential fats, manganese and tryptophan. Roast some in the oven with herbs, eat raw as a snack, stir in yoghurt, sprinkle on porridge, add to baking, smoothies and stir-fries.

Avocados - Amazing Avocados!
Eating avocados can benefit your skin, digestive health, support your heart and cholesterol health, regulate weight and reduce inflammation in arthritis. They are rich in good fats, Vitamin C and E, folate, antioxidants and potassium.

Berries – Strawberries, Raspberries, Blueberries and Blackberries pack a powerful nutritional punch! Berries help support your skin, immunity, protect against disease, assist circulation and eye health. They are rich in antioxidants, Vitamin C, folic acid, beta-carotene, potassium and folic acid. The antioxidants called Anthocyanins give berries their vibrant colour. Enjoy in smoothies; on porridge or muesli or as a snack.

Broccoli - A Nutritional Wonder! Queen of Greens. Try in stir fries, soups, salads, pasta and lightly steamed as a side. Rich in vitamins C and K, potassium, magnesium, calcium, antioxidants and zinc. Broccoli can help support bone health, digestive health, immunity, nervous and brain health, reduce skin damage and help detoxify the body. Broccoli also helps minimise the risk of disease such as cancer.

Chicken - Eat Organic or Free Range where possible. Enjoy roast, in salads, in soups, curries and stir-fries. Rich in protein, magnesium, potassium, Vitamins A and K and some B vitamins. Helps support mood, digestion, keeps energy stable, reduce mucous (think chicken soup when ill).

Coconut – Use Unrefined Organic Oil.
You can now buy chopped coconut chunks in supermarkets which are perfect for a quick snack! I use coconut oil for cooking and baking and use chunks and coconut milk in smoothies and curries. Scrambled eggs and veg cooked in coconut oil are delicious! Coconuts have a particular combination of fatty acids which benefit health, lauric acid and caprylic acid aid immunity and help destroy bacteria and viruses. Coconut products are a quick source of energy, supporting digestion and skin health, brain health and may help fat burning.

Eggs – Organic or Free Range where possible. Enjoy boiled, poached, scrambled or make scrumptious omelettes. Rich in calcium, iron, manganese, zinc, vitamin A and B vitamins, protein, and phospholipids such as choline. Antioxidants found in eggs called Lutein and Zeaxanthin support and protect your eyes. Eggs also help support good cholesterol levels, brain and mood, energy levels, immunity as well as bones and joints.

Flaxseeds / Linseeds (Ground or Whole) - Enjoy in smoothies, natural or coconut yoghurt and on porridge. Rich in calcium, magnesium, potassium, iron, B3 Omega 3 and 6 fatty acids and plant compounds called phytoestrogens. Help support digestion and stimulate gut mobility (thus helps release constipation), support heart health and female hormones.

Olives - Enjoy as a snack or in salads and casseroles. Rich in healthy fats with good levels of sodium, potassium, magnesium, iron, Vitamin E, antioxidants. Olives help support cardiovascular health, reproductive system, liver and gallbladder health, reduce anaemia and support immunity. It is also said olives are an aphrodisiac!

Onions - Enjoy in soups, casseroles, stir-fries and roasted or raw in a salad. The humble onion is rich in antioxidants and many nutrients such as vitamin C, calcium, magnesium, potassium, folic acid, sulphur, chromium and vitamin D. Onions support liver health, detoxification, and immunity. They are a natural antibiotic, as well as reducing blood clotting and high cholesterol.

Sweet Potatoes - I love this nutritious, nourishing food! Try roasting, baking, making chips or adding them to soups, stews and curries. They have plenty of fibre to help keep digestion healthy and are 'slow burn' carbs which help keep energy and blood sugar more stable. They are rich in vitamin B6 which is thought to keep heart and blood vessels healthy. Also rich in vitamin A, C, E and potassium. They also help soothe the digestive system.

Stocking Your Larder

A well-stocked cupboard and a fridge of food essentials go a long way to keeping you on track. Here are some suggestions to have on hand to help keep your food as nutritious as you can! You don't have to buy them all – see what you fancy.

Grains: brown rice, wild rice, basmati rice, oats, sugar-free muesli, quinoa, couscous, barley, wheat-free pasta, whole grain pasta, millet flakes, rice noodles.

Nuts and Seeds: walnuts, pecans, almonds, cashews, brazils; sunflower seeds, pumpkin seeds, ground flaxseeds; sugar-free nut butter: peanut, almond, cashew; tahini paste.

Beans and Lentils: lentils, chickpeas, butterbeans, borlotti beans, black-eyed peas, kidney beans, cannellini beans (dried, or tins with no added sugar).

Crackers: rye crisp bread, oatcakes, rice cakes, corn cakes.

Tins, Bottles, Cartons and Jars: Anchovies in olive oil, herring or sardines in olive oil, salmon or mackerel in brine, tuna in spring water, artichoke hearts, beetroots in brine, olives in olive oil, olive oil, walnut oil, sesame oil, coconut oil, apple cider vinegar, white wine vinegar, balsamic vinegar, mustard, honey, low sugar Thai or Indian paste, miso paste (from health food shops), tomato purée, pesto, soya sauce, lemon juice, coconut milk, chopped tomatoes, passata, sweetcorn, low sugar baked beans.

Herbs and Spices: black pepper, boullion powder, cayenne pepper, chilli flakes, cinnamon, cumin, coriander, garlic paste, ground ginger, mixed herbs, nutmeg, oregano, paprika, rosemary, sage, salt, stock cubes, thyme, turmeric, vanilla pods or essence, and seaweed flakes or strips (Nori) from health food shops.

Fridge: eggs, cheese, feta cheese, hummus, cooked meat or fish, salad leaves, fresh veg, sugar-free soya/coconut/almond milk, cows or goats milk, natural cows, sheep's or goat's yoghurt, or soya or coconut yoghurt, lemons and limes.

Freezer: fish, fruit, meat, vegetables and already cooked dishes.

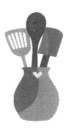

Chapter Twenty-One

PLANNING YOUR MEALS AHEAD

IT takes a little forethought, but if you schedule your meals ahead of time, you will be less tempted to swing by a take-away shop when hunger kicks in. So why not plan dinners at the start of the week; make packed lunches to take to work; have healthy nibbles at work to prevent trips to the vending machine - including nuts, seeds, dried fruit, fresh fruit, oatcakes, and even hummus; and be sure to have healthy bites in the fridge so you can throw something together at the end of a hectic day.

Simple Meal Ideas

We all get stressed, overworked, and swamped with family life, so there are bound to be times when finding time to create healthy dishes can be difficult. Enjoy the following suggestions!

Minimum Effort, Minimum Fuss for when you're tired or pushed for time.
- ✓ Baked beans (reduced sugar) and whole grain/rye toast, topped with grated goat's cheese
- ✓ Scrambled eggs with tomatoes and whole grain/rye toast
- ✓ Sardines and tomatoes and whole grain/rye toast
- ✓ Prawns with sliced avocado and lettuce, drizzled with olive oil

- ✓ Cooked mackerel, salmon or trout from the supermarket, with salad leaves, chopped cucumber and spring onions
- ✓ Smoked salmon/ hummus/goat's cheese, with oatcakes and olives
- ✓ Leftover cooked chicken and boiled potatoes, with salad
- ✓ Leftover brown rice with added tuna/salmon/smoked trout/ salmon, with sweetcorn and chopped spring onion
- ✓ Pasta with tuna, chopped tomatoes, sweetcorn and broccoli
- ✓ Tuna, tinned beans, chopped tomatoes and olive oil
- ✓ Salad with tinned beans, avocado, drizzled with lemon juice and olive oil

Meals with Benefits

Breakfast
Porridge with milk/natural yoghurt, fruit and nuts
Sugar-free muesli with milk/seeds/fruit
Oats and whole grains have good levels of B vitamins and are slow release carbs.
Boiled egg with whole grain toast or oatcake and slice avocado
Scrambled eggs with veg, e.g. tomatoes, spinach, mushrooms
Eggs are an excellent protein source to start the day and kick-start your metabolism and energy.

Smoothie with fruit, veg, seeds or nuts and milk and scoop protein powder and cinnamon
Fruit/veg/nuts and seeds are rich in vitamins, minerals and antioxidants. Cinnamon helps stabilise blood sugar levels.

Lunch (Mix & Match Lunch and Dinner)

Wholemeal sandwiches

Pitta or oatcakes with meat/fish/egg/hummus/avocado and salad

Tin mix beans/tuna with leftover brown rice and sweetcorn/salad leaves

The protein at lunchtime helps you feel fuller for longer and supports blood sugar, so you are less likely to crave sugary foods later on.

Salad with green leaves/tomatoes/radish/grated carrot/cucumber/feta/olives with added protein – turkey, tuna, beans or cottage cheese for example

Salads and veg, especially different colours have a wide range of vitamins, minerals and plant compounds beneficial for health and olives for essential fats.

Avocado and prawn salad or mackerel salad

Fish and avocado are rich in essential fats.

Homemade soups

Homemade soups are full of nutrients and nourishing for your body and mind.

Baked potato or sweet potato with a filling including reduced sugar baked beans, tuna, feta, grated mozzarella and tomato.

Potatoes have Vitamin C, some B vitamins, magnesium and potassium, while the fillings offer protein.

Dinner

Stir-fry of prawns/tofu/chicken with cashew nuts, different coloured veg and rice noodles

Omelette with veg and feta cheese and a side salad.

Whole grain or gluten free pasta with tomato based sauce, tuna, lentils and veg.

Again, plenty of veg increases your intake of valuable vitamins and minerals. Gluten free carbs (rice, rice noodles, quinoa, and sweet potato) are kinder on your digestion.
Prawns, cashews, meat and seafood are rich in the mineral zinc which is vital for immunity, hormones, reproduction, blood sugar, energy and mood.

Bean casserole, chicken casserole, beef casserole or chilli with quinoa or brown rice
Beans and lentils are an excellent source of fibre and vegetarian protein.

Good quality sausages with peas, carrots and sweet potato wedges
Vegetarian or meat curry, with plenty veg and rice
Casseroles and curries are warming and nourishing especially in autumn and winter.

Bean or homemade turkey burgers with mashed sweet potato and green veg (especially broccoli)
Kids usually love homemade burgers too!

Roast chicken with roast veg or steamed veg
Baked or grilled fish with veg and salad
Chicken is an excellent source of protein as is fish which is rich in essential fats and again veg increases intake of vitamins and minerals.

Snacks
Fruit, Nuts, Seeds
Natural / Soya / Coconut Yoghurt with Fruit, Nuts and Seeds
Chopped Veg Sticks with Dips

Nairn's Oatcakes / Rice Cakes with Hummus, Soft Cheese or Nut Butter

Olives and slice of Cheese

Coconut Chunks and a few Almonds

Apple slices with Nut Butter

Boiled egg

Dark Chocolate

Nuts

Homemade Popcorn

Atkins bars

Naked bars

Some people need to snack to support energy and blood sugar while others only need three meals but try not to snack continually throughout the day as your body needs a break from digesting food.

Choosing healthy, low sugar snacks helps you to sustain energy and has the added benefit of giving you additional vitamins and minerals.

Download my free 'Weekly Menu Planner' to help organise your family meals at: www.annecrossnutrition.co.uk

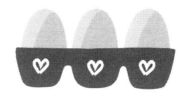

Chapter Twenty-Two

RECIPES FROM MY KITCHEN

HERE are some favourite recipes which I hope will help support your health and wellbeing and that you will also enjoy! All my own unless stated!

Scrambled Eggs

Sauté some veg - mushrooms, onion, pepper, courgette, spinach, then crumble in some feta cheese. Option: add a tsp of red pesto for extra flavour. Add 1-2 beaten eggs (with a little milk if desired). Serve with sliced avocado and/or oatcakes.

Porridge

Cook porridge oats with organic milk/sugar-free almond milk. Top with natural yoghurt, berries, walnuts/almonds.

Stewed Apples

Chop 2-3 apples. Place in a saucepan with a little water, lemon juice and a cinnamon stick (or a pinch of cinnamon powder). Cook for 10-15 mins, or until apples are soft. Option: add raisins. Eat with porridge, natural or coconut yoghurt.
Stewed apples have beneficial properties for your digestive system.

Homemade Muesli

Mix some porridge oats with quinoa (or rice flakes), chopped dried apricots, chopped almonds/brazil nuts, sunflower and pumpkin seeds.

Overnight Oats (Blueberry & Apple Bircher Muesli)

Serves 2-3

2 ½ cups/225g rolled oats (porridge oats)

1 cup/250 ml apple juice

1/3 cup/75 ml rice, almond, oat or coconut milk

½ cup/125ml natural yoghurt

Apple, cored and grated

Blueberries

Sunflower/pumpkin/linseeds – whole or ground

Put the oats in a large bowl and pour over apple juice. Cover with cling film and leave in the fridge overnight. Just before serving, stir in milk, yoghurt and grated apple. Spoon into bowls and top with blueberries, or other fruits and seeds.

Boiled Egg

Eat with an oatcake and slice of avocado/tomatoes – quick and easy!

Stock

For vegetable stock I tend to use Marigold Vegetable Bouillon, but here's my recipe for Homemade Chicken Stock: Put a chicken carcass in a large pot and cover with water. Add a chopped onion, 2-3 chopped carrots, 2-3 chopped stalks of celery, 1 tsp dried mixed herbs, salt and pepper. Cover, bring to boil and then simmer for 3-4 hours. Sieve and freeze what you don't need in freezer bags.

Green Soup
Sauté onions in a little olive oil. Add veg/chicken stock, paprika, peas, courgette, cauliflower and kale. Cook for approx 15 mins. Blend.

Orange Soup
Sauté onion in a little olive/coconut oil, add chopped carrot, cauliflower and sweet potato. Cook for approx 10 mins. Add some coconut cream (dissolved in a little water). Cook for a further 5 mins. Blend.

Butternut Squash and Kale Soup
Sauté a red onion in some olive/coconut oil, add some stock, chopped butternut squash, herbs/spices. Cook for approx 10 -12 mins. I had some kale left in my veg box so, I threw in a couple of handfuls and cooked for another 5-7 mins. Blend. It tasted surprisingly good, with a delicious sweetness coming from the butternut squash.

Homemade Guacamole
Mash 2 ripe avocados with the juice of a lemon into a paste. Add ½ a red onion finely chopped. Add one large tomato finely chopped. Season with salt and black pepper. That's it! Enjoy on oatcakes, whole grain crackers, or with veg sticks.

Cucumber Boats with Yoghurt, Walnuts and Feta Cheese
Slice a cucumber in half lengthwise. Smother with natural yoghurt or soft cheese. Top with crumbled feta cheese and walnuts. Cut into pieces for a healthy snack.

Cauliflower Hummus
(Lovely on oatcakes, whole grain pitta, or with veg sticks)

Take a whole cauliflower head, cut into florets and place on a baking tray. Drizzle with approx 2 tbsps olive oil, salt and pepper. Cover with foil and cook for approx 12 mins until beginning to soften. Remove foil and cook for another 10 mins. Turn florets and cook 10 more mins until starting to brown. Blend with 2 tbsps Tahini plus 1 tbsp lemon juice and 1 crushed garlic clove. Add a little more olive oil or water for a thinner consistency if desired.

Cauliflower Rice

Take several florets of cauliflower and whiz in a food processor. Stir fry in some olive or coconut oil with some veg - onions, mushrooms, peppers and carrots. Add a little soya sauce if desired at the end of cooking. Cook till veg softens. Serve with beans, meat or fish. You can also buy cauliflower rice in supermarkets. Low carb and delicious!

Sweet Potato Wedges

Chop sweet potato into wedges or chunks, drizzle with olive/coconut oil. Add herbs/chilli flakes. Bake for approx 20 mins, or until cooked.

Smoked Mackerel and Avocado Pâté

225g/8oz smoked mackerel fillets skinned, 2oz low fat soft cheese, 1 ripe avocado, some lemon juice and black pepper. Mix all ingredients until smooth or in a food processor. Serve with oatcakes and salad leaves. The good fats in this pâté are beneficial for your skin, hair, hormones, brain, joints and heart.

Tuna (or Chickpeas) and Feta Simple Salad

Put some salad leaves in a bowl. Mix drained tinned tuna, feta cheese, chopped tomato, chopped cucumber, chopped red or spring onion, and olives. Add to salad leaves. Drizzle olive oil and balsamic vinegar onto the salad and mix.

You could add some pine nuts or walnuts for good fats. Use chickpeas if you don't eat tuna.

Quinoa Salad

Take ½ cup uncooked quinoa (keen-wah) and cook in a cup of chicken or veg stock for approx 15mins. Drain any excess liquid. Mix in olive oil, crumbled feta cheese, lemon juice and chopped spring onion or chopped roasted veg.

Wild Salmon Pasta

Cook some whole grain or wheat-free pasta and drain. Mix in cooked salmon, peas, cauliflower and baby tomatoes. Sprinkle with a little grated cheese. Sophia loves this!

Turkey Burgers

In a food processor whizz 1tsp tomato sauce or purée with ½ a grated carrot and ½ a grated courgette, and a little flour. Put mixture in a bowl with a pack of turkey mince and shape into small burgers. Dust with a little flour and put in the fridge to harden a little. Braise gently on a low heat in olive or coconut oil turning once. Serve with sweet potato wedges and some steamed green veg. Option: Mix in feta/zest of lime and 1 tbsp chopped fresh coriander. Note: A pack of mince makes approx 10 small burgers.

One Pot Turkey Meal (Beef/Quorn/Green Lentil/Beans)

In a large pan lightly brown a pack of turkey mince in coconut or olive oil over a low heat until nearly cooked. Add chopped carrot, sweet potatoes, orange or yellow pepper, courgette, and mushrooms. Add some spices - cumin, turmeric, coriander and paprika. Add stock and a tin of chopped tomatoes (also a small tin of kidney beans or chickpeas if desired). Simmer for approx 30 mins. You can also substitute grass fed, organic or regular beef mince, Quorn mince, green lentils, or beans.

Homemade Chicken Nuggets

Cut some chicken breasts into slices. Dip into beaten egg. Whizz up a couple of slices of bread in a food processor to make bread crumbs and coat the chicken and egg mixture with the bread crumbs. Bake in the oven for approx 18 mins. Serve with steamed veg and potatoes. Adults and kids alike can enjoy.

Chicken and Lentils

Brown some chicken thighs or chopped chicken breasts in olive or coconut oil for a couple of minutes. Add chopped onion and stir. Put approx 800ml boiled water in a jug with some bouillon powder, ½ tsp of powdered coriander, ½ tsp ground turmeric, ½ tsp of paprika, ½ tsp ginger OR add a big spoonful of Balti paste. Add liquid and to the chicken and onions. Add chopped carrot and yellow pepper. Cook for approx 15 mins before adding a small cup of red lentils. Cook for a further 15-20 mins. You may find you need to add a little more water. Enjoy with rice or a side salad.

Thai Red/Yellow Curry (Chicken/Prawn/Chickpea/Tofu)

Chop 2 chicken breasts and cook on a low heat for a few minutes in some coconut or olive oil. Add chopped red pepper, orange pepper, sweet potato, and cauliflower florets. Mix a little veg stock, half a jar of Thai red or yellow paste and a little water and add to the pan. Simmer for approx 30-35 mins until chicken and veg are tender. Add a tin of coconut milk, spinach leaves or pak choi and simmer for another 5 mins. Serve with rice or rice noodles. You could use prawns, chickpeas or tofu instead.

Cauliflower Dahl

from the low GL Cookbook by Patrick Holford

2 onions diced

2 cloves of garlic crushed

¾ inch fresh root ginger peeled and chopped

½ tsp turmeric

½ tsp ground cumin

¼ tsp cayenne pepper

2tbsp coconut oil or olive oil

75g/3oz red lentils

1pint water

2tsp Marigold vegetable bullion powder

Third of a medium sized cauliflower cut into florets

Put the onions, garlic and spices into a blender and purée. Heat the oil in a pan and add the purée mixture and fry gently for approx 5 mins. Add the water, lentils and bouillon powder to the pan and boil for 10mins. Add the cauliflower, cover and simmer for 15 mins to allow the lentils to cook down and the cauliflower to soften.

Tomato and Butter Bean Stew

1 big can chopped tomatoes (440gms)

1 big tin butter beans (440gms)

2 sliced leeks

1 tbsp veg stock

Chopped veg of choice (onion, carrot, courgette, peppers)

Sauté leeks and onion in a little olive oil and the stock for approx 5 mins. Add chopped tomatoes, butter beans, chopped veg and simmer for approx 10-15 mins. Season with pepper and dried or fresh mixed herbs (parsley, thyme, coriander). Serve with brown rice or quinoa and a small green salad.

Slow Cooking is a great way to make warming and nourishing stews and casseroles during the winter months. It saves time and the food is ready when you come home from work. There are many recipes available online, but here are two I particularly enjoy making. You can also bulk out the recipe by adding butterbeans or chickpeas and I usually make enough to last a couple of meals:

Chicken Stew

Place chicken thighs (free range or organic if possible) in the slow cooker with chopped red and yellow peppers, onion, courgette, sweet or regular potato, and carrot. Add a little stock and a chicken 'stock pot'. Cook on low for approx 6-7 hours.

Beef Stew

Chop stewing steak (or buy it already chunked). Add onions, leeks, carrots, sweet potatoes, peppers, mushrooms and most of a tin of chopped tomatoes. Add a little stock and a beef 'stock pot'. Cook on low for approx 6-7 hours. The meat becomes really tender having released its collagen and other nutrients – which helps support bones, joints, skin and ligaments. Serve on its own or with a little rice and green veg.

Smoothie

Blend chia seeds soaked for approx 10 mins with 1 scoop whey or other protein powder, ½ ripe avocado, ½ ripe pear, a handful of kale and unsweetened almond milk. Yum! I usually have my smoothies after a session at the gym or a dance class.

Sticky Energy Balls

¼ cup finely grated carrot

¼ cup rolled oats

¼ cup raisins

¼ cup sunflower seeds

¼ cup wheat germ

1 tbsp honey

3 tbsps peanut or almond or other nut butter

Mix, roll into balls and coat in desiccated coconut, if desired.

Ice Lollies

There are many combinations, but we often make them with apple juice, a small spoon of natural yoghurt and a selection of chopped fruit - apple, banana, strawberries, pineapple etc. Freeze overnight in ice lolly holders. Even better when it is warm and sunny!

IN CONCLUSION

My Top Health Tips

Eat Real Food

Nourish Yourself

Move

Exercise

Smell The Roses

Breathe

Relax

Take Time Out

Be Kind to Yourself

Love and Laugh

Slow Down from Time to Time

Find Enjoyment in What You Do!

A Poem (written in the midst of anxiety!)

The mind can be crazy
And can cause us some distress.
Low mood or depression,
Or like me, an anxiety mess!

Our thoughts go over and over
And often we are not aware.
Start to become more conscious
To acknowledge the thoughts that are there.

It's no easy task
Releasing negative mind chatter,
But there are techniques and tips
To show you truly matter.

The true you, the most beautiful,
Is there deep inside.
The diamond, the love
That a worried mind hides.

Don't try to control or judge your thoughts
Or focus on them, that makes them grow!
Just acknowledge, accept
And let them gently onward flow

Flow on by, on a river or cloud,
Or challenge, perhaps as CBT taught
It's just your ego speaking.
Or simply choose a nicer thought!

If you, like me,
Fear feeling stuck
Know healthy food and exercise
Can soon break up the muck!

Try to find an occupation
That re-focuses your worried mind.
For some its arts and puzzles,
Gardening, music! Whatever you can find!

Try grounding with an energy skill.
Focus energy in hands, legs and feet.
Stomping and star jumps release tension
And take away the heat!

Self-compassion and gratitude ease,
Focus on beautiful things.
Try not to always rush ahead.
Stay in the present - so much peace it brings.

Put your hand on your heart,
Ask your soul to guide.
Ask for love, ease and peace
And stay on your own amazing side.

Deep breathing and meditation
Stills a mind that's racing fast
Connecting with our inner knowing
Can release fears from the past.

If symptoms of discomfort come
Accept, relax, release
As are bodies are rebalancing
It helps to bring more peace.

Keep going!
Onward on your journey, little steps at a time.
Ask your guides and angels to empower you
And everything will work out fine.

HELPFUL RESOURCES

Websites

www.ausflowers.com
Flower Essences & Organic Skin & Body Care

www.anneholisticnutrition.co.uk
Practical, sound, effective nutritional advice to take into your daily life

www.bant.org.uk
British Association of Nutritional Therapists - Professional Body with details of how to contact a therapist and how to train as one

www.faithinnature.co.uk
Hair, Skin Care plus Washing & Laundry Products

www.greenpeople.co.uk
Organic Body, Hair & Skin Care Products

www.heartmath.org/com/co.uk
Courses, Services and Products to help reduce stress, enhance life, boost resistance - "helping activate the heart of humanity"

www.heart2shine.com
Flower Essences, Courses and Energy Healing to help your heart shine

www.naturalfoodbenefits.com
Describing the Health Benefits of Natural Foods

www.self-compassion.org
Dr Kristen Neff guided loving kindness meditations and more – see also her YouTube talks and tips

www.whfoods.com
Helping you eat and cook the world's healthiest foods for optimal health

Books

Lorna Byrne	A Message of Hope from the Angels
Paul Gilbert	The Compassionate Mind
Marilyn Glenville	Getting Pregnant Faster *boost your fertility in 3 months*
Kyle Gray	Raise your Vibration & Angel Prayers
Tracey Hogg	The Baby Whisperer
Patrick Holford	The Optimum Nutrition Bible
Christiane Northrup MD	Women`s Bodies, Women`s Wisdom *creating physical and emotional health and healing*
S Orsillo & L Roemer	The Mindful Way Through Anxiety
John C Parkin	F**k It
Candace Pert	Molecules of Emotion *why you feel the way you feel*
Trudeau R Peterson	Nurturing the soul of your family *10 ways to reconnect and find peace in everyday life*
Eckhart Tolle	Practicing the Power of Now *A guide to spiritual enlightenment*
James Wilson	Adrenal Fatigue the 21st century stress syndrome *what it is and how you can recover*

ACKNOWLEDGEMENTS

Thanks to my wonderful friends both old and new who accept, love and believe in me.

To some amazing people/therapists who have helped me on my journey over the years: Dr Mason Brown, Zoe, Shirley and Jacqui from Heart to Shine, May Anderson, Patrick Harding and Heather Boyd. Thank you also to Angie Cameron for introducing me to the concept of self-compassion.

Thanks to the clients, workshop participants and students I work with who continue to help me learn, grow and enable me to share my knowledge of the powerful benefits of food.

Thank you to Angela Clarence – editor extraordinaire! for all your help with editing, and the whole publishing process.

Thank you to Cassia Friello for your beautiful images, ideas and colours which have helped bring my book to life.

Thank you to Geoff Fisher for your skill and knowledge in taking my words and text and making them ready for print!

Finally, thanks to all those before me who have written books with the primary purpose of sharing knowledge, understanding and helping others.

21108892R00075

Printed in Great Britain
by Amazon